ACCEPTING DESTINY

Praise for *Accepting Destiny*

"Isabelle Morton is a treasure. So few teachers of practical energy medicine are as genuinely heartfelt and compassionate as Isabelle. Her information and methods source directly from her visits with inner-world Guides on the subtle planes of our Earth, and her work is completely unique in the world of energetic healing. Isabelle's teachings on Gemstone Therapy have opened up limitless possibilities for me as an energetic healer, for myself as well as my clients. Moreover, Isabelle encourages her students to become their own teachers, and to learn directly from the gemstones themselves. Read her story and be inspired!"

—Robyn Arrington, MSW,
Gemstone Therapy Practitioner

"Witness the glorious gift of a whole new level of gemstone medicine, offering us innovative techniques to diagnose and treat complex, debilitating medical conditions in today's ever-changing environment. This is a toolkit that brings together a rare combination of both safety and intense power, rocketing it to the forefront of innovations supporting health on all levels of being."

—Cari Nyland, ND, DAFNS, GTP

"Isabelle Morton and her work have an elegant quality and unlimited potential. Working with her I have experienced tremendous growth and healing on numerous levels. I can't imagine life without support from the Mineral Kingdom and Isabelle's magnificent talents and tools. Isabelle, thank you for the treasure you are and the treasures you've shared and introduced to me."

—Barbara K.

"I believe that the Gemstone Therapy Institute that Isabelle founded in 2009 will serve to elevate Gemstone Energy Medicine to its rightful place alongside homeopathy and acupuncture as a complete, holistic healing system and modality, for self-therapy and practitioners. As a Gemstone Therapy Practitioner certified by Isabelle and the Gemstone Therapy Institute, I have been privileged to share this work with hundreds of clients and students who in turn have shared their experiences with others. Isabelle's leadership, personal example, and love are a testament to her commitment to this work and to humanity. She is an inspiration to us all."

—Herbert Wheeler, BSMT, GTP

"Gemstone Therapy has increased my awareness of all that the earth has to offer for nourishment and support. I find the gemstone necklaces support me in changes I want to make, ground me when I need grounding and provide emotional support when that is needed. My life is enhanced by using gemstones—and they're beautiful to wear as well!"

—R. M.

"I was going through very bad phase in my life and was asking the universe to help me out. I found Isabelle. She has an amazing ability to view and work with our energy bodies. She works mostly with energy chakras. She corrects their shape, orientation, color and also frees them from unwanted energies using the healing power of gemstones. I was amazed by Isabelle's ability to correctly identify the cause of the issue and thereafter fixing the same. I am ever grateful and thankful to Isa and the universe for bringing this healing into my life."

—K.M.

"I have been on a healing journey for years and years trying to find healing work that works for me and the right practitioners with whom I feel comfortable and who really know what they are doing. I have spent thousands and thousands of dollars and worked with dozens of practitioners, mostly with temporary or meager results. A lot of the issues I have sought help for are from experiencing overwhelming amounts of trauma and injury in this lifetime.

"Finally, I have found someone who truly understands what has happened to my body and why things are the way they are now. I have never been able to get anyone else to understand that.

"Isabelle works from a deeply rooted knowingness about the gemstones and how to use them and is providing me with the healing I have long sought. During sessions it feels as though she and the gemstones are one and totally devoted to me. I am seeing my issues resolve and believe that gemstone therapy is key to recovering and maintaining my health from now on."

—R.E.

"Many years ago I discovered therapeutic gemstones and gemstone therapy as a healing modality. It was the first approach I used, including mainstream medicine, which really improved my life. Since then it has consistently been one of the most effective tools I have for improving my health. I also receive such feelings of love and support from my experiences with gemstone healing and I love how there is a correlation between how beautiful they are and how effectively they improve my life. Isabelle, it's wonderful how you're adding to this field."

—Karen Kolczak

"I have found Gemstone and Diamond Therapy to be profound and life-changing for me, my family, and clients over these many years of working with this incredible healing modality."

—Linda Lile, Ph.D., GTP, ABD

"For me, working with Isabelle's unique gemstone protocols and applications is a breath of fresh air! The gemstones have offered a dimension of healing in my life like nothing else. I have learned so much from her in her trainings through the Gemstone Therapy Institute and am forever grateful to her for bringing this incredible modality into the world."

—Barbara D., PT

"Isabelle Morton has developed a system of healing that has helped me learn about myself, given me direction, and helped me to heal old wounds and patterns. Her ability to work with me at my current level as well as her innate sense of who I am incorporates the meaning of a true healer. Isabelle's knowledge of gemstone systems is powerful and by far exemplary in the ability to heal. Definitely life-changing."

—Melissa Nemeth

"Gemstone Therapy helped my emotional trauma and my physical condition to stabilize and rebalance after my husband passed from a heart attack. It was invaluable. This therapy continues to provide me harmony and gentle guidance as well as opening me to levels of my individual energetic and human potential. I am grateful. Isabelle, thank you for providing the platform for gemstone and diamond therapies. I have great respect for your knowledge and commitment and for the diamond and gemstone gifts so lovingly provided by Spirit."

—Jeanie Morrissey

"Gemstone Therapy was a complete surprise that changed my life. I am able to receive nourishment every day from the gemstones. After working with Isabelle and the gemstones, I have received such beautiful guidance to go within to find great sources of understanding, happiness, and peace. I truly will never be able to wear any other jewelry in this lifetime!!"

—J.L., GTP

"I've found Gemstone Therapy to be all encompassing. It has helped me gain a deeper self-awareness and given me tools to address health concerns as well. I love the self-help aspect of gemstone therapy. Thank you Isa for being courageous and bringing this unique modality into the world!"

—Luba Lischynsky

"I had the good fortune to be introduced to Isabelle through her books when she was known under a different name. They inspired a leap into using gemstone necklaces and spheres when I didn't even wear jewelry. I do believe it changed my life, facilitating growth and supporting all of my endeavors. I was then again fortunate to encounter her when she started GEMFormulas.

"The gemstones, the diamonds, the Guardians and Isabelle are an important part of my life. Isabelle's knowledge, skill and partnership with the Guardians are remarkable and benefits us all. I am certainly stronger, healthier and happier from these experiences. And I am grateful to Isabelle for her sessions and training which have allowed me to grow, heal, and contribute to others as well. Thank you Isa!"

—D.M., GTP

"Isa is an energetic surgeon and a gifted genius. It is truly remarkable how she ushers in Gemstone Therapy with creditability and sophistication. I have always felt grounded and supported by the gemstones in every aspect of my life and over 25 years of study, I've always know in my heart of hearts this is a true 21st Century healing modality. I am deeply and profoundly grateful that Isabelle has brought this modality to the world. If I were to choose one word for gemstone therapy, it would be upliftment—mind, body and soul."

—Stephanie O'Dell, Certified
Gemstone Therapy practitioner

"Isabelle's teachings have allowed me to learn the art of gentle inquiry, listening, trusting in the reply to the inquiry that is freely offered by the gemstones and the Gemstone Guardians. This process has become a paramount element in my life, work with the gems, and in my professional work as a Certified Rolfer.® Who would have imagined even the possibility of such profound experiences from a strand of beautiful gems????"

—Harriet O.

"I've learned a lot about myself and the possibilities which are available to everyone with diamond therapy. Isabelle's skills, understanding, and abilities offered me a gradual acquaintance with gemstones and their unique benefits. Every session contributed deeper and more far reaching benefits than ever before. I felt like a different person and yet more intimately familiar with myself. Not only that but I liked *me* in a way that I wasn't showing up before. How about that? I'm still amazed! The best part is that the whole process is a lot of fun, *a lot of fun!* Where has this been all my life?"

—J.W.

"Gemstone Therapy has taken me on a journey of self-discovery. Most notably, I am learning a great deal about being a multi-dimensional being. The gems have taught me to look beyond the surface, and beyond physicality, where there are keys to open doors to the other levels of cause. This work has completely changed the way I look at life, at the body, and all my relationships!

"Isabelle is giving us the tools and the methods to explore the Science of the Human Energy Field in ways that are precise, defined, and transformative. The protocols she is teaching are revolutionary and will change the way we look at psychology and medicine in a very short time. I am honored and privileged to be her student at the Gemstone Therapy Institute

"As a certified Gemstone Therapy practitioner, I can't wait to contribute to the body of research! From the deepest part of my being, thank you Isabelle!"

—Debra Lucero Kraft, MA, NBCT, GTP

"Isabelle Morton is a very special seer. I have been using gems for balancing, healing, and enhancing consciousness for 46 years. Gems are tools bridging the gap between pure consciousness and the subtle qualities of the mind and body. It's like the un-manifested nurturing sap in a flower coming up to manifest beautiful colors and vibrations. Isabelle Morton's knowledge of gems and her nurturing patience has touched my heart deeply."

—Gordon P.

"Before I found GEMFormulas and had gemstone sessions with Isabelle Morton I felt I needed to move forward but wasn't clear about what my purpose was or how to figure it out. Isabelle worked with me remotely using gemstones to clear away the confusion. The sessions were gentle but very effective. We addressed the core of the blockages and cleared them. A benefit of the gemstone sessions is that it has allowed me to discover what my heart is really calling out to do. I am now feeling confident that I am beginning a new career with a bright future. I am very grateful!"

—B.L.

"It has been a fascinating journey studying and working with Isabelle Morton. Isabelle has an amazing gift and a mission to share her knowledge of gemstones and how they can assist us in our health and well-being. We have learned a lot about therapeutic gemstones, how our physical health and well-being is deeply connected to our energetic health, and how to utilize these beautiful and precious gemstones for ourselves and in our gemstone therapy practice. The best part is wondering where this journey will take us next!"

—Marjorie Hill and Gary Wright
Certified Gemstone Therapy
Practitioners

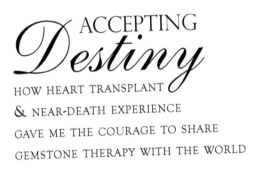

ACCEPTING *Destiny*

HOW HEART TRANSPLANT
& NEAR-DEATH EXPERIENCE
GAVE ME THE COURAGE TO SHARE
GEMSTONE THERAPY WITH THE WORLD

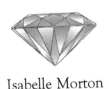

Isabelle Morton

GEMFormulas LLC
Manchester, Connecticut

Accepting Destiny

Isabelle Morton

Copyright © 2016 by Isabelle Morton

Printed in the U.S.A.

ISBN: 978-0-9849967-3-5

Edited by Mary Carroll Moore

Designed by Robin McBride

Cover photo: Fadil Berisha *www.fadilberisha.com*

Library of Congress Control Number: 2016904682
GEMFormulas LLC
PO Box 4065
Manchester, Connecticut U.S.A. 06045

www.isabellemorton.com
www.GEMFormulas.com

Dedicated to
My donor family with love and gratitude.
Thank you for giving me a second chance.

and

To all who love healing
with diamonds and gemstones,
for making my life meaningful.

CONTENTS

NOTE TO READER

*T*his book is a memoir and is based on true events, people, and situations as I recall them. However some names, biographical data, and other minor details have been changed, conflated, or omitted. These insignificant alterations do not impact the essential truth of my story. The conversations all come from my recollections. They are not written to represent word-for-word transcripts. Rather, I have retold them in a way that evokes the feeling and meaning of what was said, and, in all instances, the essence of the dialogue is accurate.

1

TIME TO GET BACK ON TRACK

*O*ne's destiny, if it offers something positive and uplifting to others, should be something one wants to achieve—not to struggle against. For ten years I had denied my gifts and ignored my life's purpose. Apparently, it had been long enough.

The morning of October 22, 2002, I awoke with the terrible conviction that my life was about to get back on track. The memories of a prophetic dream were fresh in my awareness. I scrambled for my journal to write them down. No need to turn on the bedside lamp—the morning sun was streaming through the open window into my small bedroom along with a crisp autumn breeze.

I grabbed a pen and refocused on remembering my dream. The moan of my neighbor's leaf-blower was beginning to distract me.

"It's time to start..." I wrote.

Sheaves of the dream began to disappear into the abyss of forgetfulness.

"thinking about..."

I reached deeply for the next phrase. A favorite author of mine once compared remembering a dream to trying to catch a slippery fish.

"changing your H _ _ _ _."

What was that last word?

It had vanished.

I fell back into bed, trying my hardest to remember anything beyond that one solitary line. Some big change was about to happen. Maybe I could avoid it—if only I knew the identity of the five-letter word that began with the letter "H."

I checked the clock. I was living alone with my daughter, four-year-old Kellan, the youngest of my five children. She was still asleep in the next room. It was time to wake her up.

Bob, whom I'd been dating for two years, would be here any minute to help me pack my car. We were planning a four-hour trip to my mother's house where we would drop off Kellan. The following morning we would fly to Minneapolis to attend a spiritual seminar. The seminar was celebrating the upcoming year of spiritual healing—a topic that was to have special meaning for me in the next twelve hours.

I wished the letter H might have stood for husband. Oh well, too many letters.

"What's the rush?" Bob would say when I broached the subject of an engagement. "I've already been married, and you've been divorced—twice."

Five kids with two different fathers, a nearly empty bank account, and a writing career that was barely supporting me—my life was complicated. Still, a committed relationship was important to me. Of course, I didn't want to tell Bob about the strong premonition I'd had as a teenager. My true purpose in life would only be fulfilled when I was married. At age forty-one, I wanted to get on with my life, and I believed I needed Bob to do that.

"Maybe the dream is telling me I should sell my house," I said to him as I made room in the trunk for our suitcases and Kellan's things. Bob was a decade older than me, blue-eyed, well-muscled, and handsome in his gray hair. What I liked most about him was his dedication to spirituality. This man walked the talk. He had the kindest of hearts and old-fashioned values, but when it came to making a long-term commitment to our relationship, he was one of the most stubborn people I knew.

Bob grabbed his bag from his minivan, which he had parked in my double-wide driveway. "If it was my dream, it would mean it was time to change my horse."

"You don't have a horse."

"For me, a horse is a vehicle. Maybe you need a new car."

What is it with guys and cars?

I reached within myself for a sense of rightness and didn't find it. "I don't think my dream means that."

Bob began piecing our piles of stuff into the trunk.

"It could be homes," I said carefully.

"Or it could be humor."

"Very funny." I handed him Kellan's stroller.

The symptoms began that night. Bob and I were cuddling in my mom's sofa bed in the den watching baseball. The Giants were playing the Angels in the fifth game of the World Series. Suddenly the peace I was enjoying was replaced with a flash-flood of adrenaline from hell.

I sprang out of bed.

"Are you okay?"

"I don't know."

I couldn't catch my breath. My body felt as though I had just received intravenously the equivalent of twenty cups of espresso, or as though my insides were being shaken like salt. Was this what it felt like to jump from an airplane attached to a bungee cord?

"I think I'm going to be sick."

3

I had barely enough strength to make it the few steps through the laundry room to the small bathroom, where I repeatedly went to empty my digestive tract.

Where was my strength?

I thought I was perfectly healthy. I worked full time, attended karate classes, and was an active volunteer at our temple. I also took care of Kellan and her sister AriaRay, who was twenty months older, and who was presently with her dad—ex-husband number two.

To calm down I practiced chanting HU, which is a favorite mantra, and I called on my spiritual guide for help. I tried tai chi, yoga, chi gung, and even Lamaze natural childbirth breathing techniques. Nothing seemed to help. Later I learned these activities may have saved my life.

I used natural and alternative healing methods because I was comfortable with them. In the late 1980s, I had played a major role in bringing out a modality called Gemstone Therapy, which was based on crystals made into spheres and worn as necklaces. At my first divorce, I stepped away from my work and gave up all my copyrights, sure I would never return.

While therapeutic gemstones are not typically used in acute situations like the one I was experiencing, had I still been working with them, I certainly would have reached for them for support. I would have chosen from among those I would have brought with me. These days, I always travel with several.

A gemstone necklace would have provided comfort. It could have balanced and steadied my energies, and lifted my vibrations enough so that I might not have felt so exhausted during the ordeal. Or it may have opened my awareness so that I might have recognized what was going on and called 911—before I lost consciousness.

Fortunately, two hours after the nightmarish feelings overcame me, they simply vanished. All was well again, although I felt as tired as an old dishrag. We attributed it to a stomach bug and went to bed.

At four o'clock in the morning, the caffeine buzz started up again. I tried to calm myself back to sleep.

"Just relax. Reee-laaaaax," I repeated to myself.

My body had other ideas. A survival instinct forced me out of bed and back to the toilet. There was nothing left to come out.

I endured another ninety minutes of hell. And then, as though a switch was flipped, I was suddenly overcome by:

Deep.

Pervading.

Peace.

Bob found me sprawled on the laundry room floor, drooling.

"Isa?" He shook my shoulder. I didn't hear him.

"Isabelle!"

When I did not respond, he called 911 and then ran up to my mom's room to wake her and tell her what was going on.

Meanwhile, I was now pain free and enveloped by a gray mist. It was accompanied by the deepest, thickest, richest Peace—of the sort I never could have imagined possible. After all I had been through in the past few hours, the peace was oh, so welcome.

The blue luminescent form of my spiritual guide glowed in my peripheral vision. Another time I might have been curious about the closeness and reality of his company. Right now, although his presence was reassuring, after what I'd just endured, the peace was all that mattered.

A light on the horizon called to me, and yet I had no interest in it, nor of exploring the strange world in which I found myself. All I wanted to do was to be left undisturbed. I wanted to relish and luxuriate in this most profound sense of serenity. The gray world had become my Peaceful Place, and I could have stayed there forever.

Too soon, off in the distance, I heard an unfamiliar male voice trying to get my attention. He kept distracting me from the Peace.

The voice was annoying. Like a pesky housefly.

"What's the name of our President?"

The question made no sense.

I struggled to place the question inside my reality and could not. It did not belong in this world. I had read about the sun worlds and the moon worlds, which lay just before the bright worlds of true heavenly light. I guessed this was where I was, somewhere just outside of heaven. I looked on the horizon for the light and the gateway to something higher and brighter. A part of me longed for that light, and I felt as though I was moving closer to it.

"What's the name of our President?" The distracting voice drew me back.

Reluctantly, I opened one eye and saw a black, well-polished shoe a few inches from my nose. "Hmm, steel-toed," I thought. "Bob doesn't wear shoes like that."

I became aware that I was horizontal, cold, and that the entrance hall of my mom's house was filled with strangers. The washing machine loomed overhead.

"Who is our President?"

I tried desperately to ignore the distraction. I shut my eye and did my best to return to the thick blanket of peace. Meanwhile my mind tried to remember who had won the last election.

"Ask me another question," I murmured.

"She's back," the paramedic announced, and I was lifted onto a gurney. I insisted on giving Kellan a hug goodbye and assured her I was all right.

As they locked the ambulance door behind me, I knew my year of spiritual healing had begun. I hadn't a clue how deep the healing would actually be—nor that it would help me rediscover my passion for working with healing gemstones.

2

HOW MY GEMSTONE JOURNEY BEGAN

y gemstone journey began one cold Colorado evening in 1987. I was getting ready to turn in for the night when I heard my then husband call out in pain. I found him doubled over on the bare wood floor of our spacious and nearly empty bedroom.

We were renting a home in the shadow of the Rocky Mountains. We had moved from Tucson, where I graduated college, to Boulder, then to Kauai, back to Tucson, and then back to Boulder—all within five years. We didn't have much furniture.

"It's my leg," David said.

I helped him onto the bed. "What happened?"

"The pain—it came out of nowhere. Again."

"Do you want to go to the emergency room?"

"They can't help me."

He was right. We had been down this road before with other pain that David had experienced and the doctors had scoffed at us. If we went to the emergency room, they would give my husband pain killers, and then they would tell him to go see a psychiatrist.

I turned up the thermostat in the bedroom to help make David feel more comfortable.

"Is there anything I can do?" I was thinking of hot compress-es. Maybe some tea. "Would some gentle massage help?"

He said touch was painful.

Then he said, "I've heard of an energy worker who releases pain by unzipping the skin. Would you try that?"

His request took me aback. I knew he didn't mean actually opening his body, only making an energetic portal for the pain to come out. Nonetheless, unzipping people sounded "psychic." I wanted nothing to do with anything psychic for fear it would draw me away from true spirituality. Besides, I was skeptical it could work.

I left the bedroom to get a hot compress and some ice. May-be one or the other would help.

Both made the pain worse. David began to feel desperate. "You've got to try. There's nothing else we can do."

Was there?

I looked at our reflection in the sliding glass door that sep-arated us from the black night. Was this really our only hope?

Unfortunately, I sensed it was. Somehow it felt like the right thing to do.

Inwardly, I declared that whatever I did was for the good of the whole, and I would do it in God's name. Then I put aside my concerns about psychic traps and pulled up a chair to posi-tion myself beside David's leg.

I thought of what a zipper looked like, and touched my fin-gertips to a point on David's leg above the pain. Intuitively, I drew open the zipper by running my fingertips along an imagi-nary line over the pain to a point near his ankle. Then, I repo-sitioned my fingers at the middle of this line and gently spread open the energetic tissue I had unzipped.

"Good God," I said. To my utter amazement, I could see inside his leg and the source of the pain was unmistakable. "It looks like a long metal blade, like a sword."

"Take it out."

"I can't." It was deeply embedded and worse, I also saw various types of ugly energies dripping out and also rising up like fog out of the opening I had made. Inside were patches of black tar and what appeared to be pools of thick dark blood. David's leg had become an energetic mess, and I hadn't a clue how to clean it up.

Meanwhile, his agony increased.

Inwardly I beseeched my spiritual guide for assistance. "Please help me," I said inwardly, though I may have said the words aloud, too.

I felt a presence behind me that was so strong I actually turned to look. There before me stood a benevolent being dressed in brown. He looked very much like a monk of medieval times and somehow I knew that he was a healer.

"David," I whispered, "You won't believe this, but an inner guide has just appeared."

"Who is he?"

"I'm a doctor and I can help you," the monk confirmed telepathically. I relayed the message to David.

"How?" I asked in my thoughts.

He sent me images of healing techniques he could use.

At the time, I didn't know that he could have provided this assistance directly. Or that he could have guided me to do the work myself. I thought I needed to channel him. Channeling is the process of allowing an otherworldly being to occupy your body and use your voice, and also sometimes your hands and eyes, to communicate and operate in the physical world. At the time, it was the only way I knew that non-physical beings could interact with physical ones.

So, necessary or not, I invited him in.

Instantly I felt him slip into my body and take control. To allow him work on David, I stepped aside by moving out of my body. I had no idea I could do this. I just did it. From a vantage point behind my shoulder, I could see both David and the doctor. At the same time, I could observe what the doctor was doing.

I saw him summon crystalline decanters of colored liquids that appeared on glass trays, just when he needed to pour them into David's wound. Somehow I recognized they contained gem-stone energies. Other instruments also came into view—things I'd never seen before. He used compresses, draining tubes, tiny siphons, and geometric containment fields. He used all his tools deftly and proficiently.

It was odd to have someone else move my hands and operate my voice; otherwise, channeling the monk did not hurt or feel strange. Any misgivings I may have had were overcome by a strong feeling of certainty and empowerment. This doctor knew exactly what was wrong and how to fix it. His confidence was assuring.

"You're going to be all right," he said to David, using my voice.

David watched me work—rather he saw my hands moving. While I could see the tools being used, I was sure they were physically invisible. I couldn't imagine what David must have been thinking, and yet he took it all in stride.

At one point, the doctor asked for some of the gemstone sphere necklaces David and I had been collecting. We had been in the fine diamond and estate jewelry business for several years, and had our store up for sale. The semi-precious beads had a special appeal, and we planned to start a new business around them.

"I could bring them in energetically," the doctor said, "but physical tissues require physical tools."

David told him where we kept the box of gems, and using my body, he got up to get them. First he got out a strand of Frosted Quartz spheres and asked David to hold them on his leg. Their energies brought in a beautiful white light, with a soft gentle glow, that surrounded David's leg. I could see this energy soothe and heal.

The doctor took out the Emerald beads and, holding both ends of the strand, gently ran the necklace up David's leg repeatedly. I watched how the Emerald energies neutralized most of the ugly energies, which simply dissipated. He used the Dark Green Aventurine spheres in a similar way to help the cells release their hold on these unwanted energies. He coordinated the application of the physical gems with his colorful gemstone liquids.

Then he removed the sword and handed it to an assistant— an angel-like being—who appeared just in time. He and the doctor exchanged a nod of gratitude, and the angel took the sword away.

The doctor selected Blue Sapphire and this time held it above the leg. "To help reorganize the tissues," he explained.

Soon the wound in David's energy-body repaired, and the ugly energies cleared away. The physical tissues inside his leg looked almost perfectly healthy.

"How are you feeling now?" the doctor asked, again using my voice.

"The pain is much better."

The doctor showed us how to use the strands of Dark Green Aventurine and Frosted Quartz as compresses to further the healing process. He hinted at their therapeutic value when worn as necklaces, too.

"Wearing gemstone necklaces has therapeutic value?" David asked.

"Most certainly. The Dark Green Aventurine will help the cells continue to detoxify, and the Frosted Quartz will bring in healing light that will help balance the energies in your leg."

Then the doctor turned his attention to me. Telepathically, he communicated that the use of the gemstones during David's healing session had been observed by a Healing Council. If I wanted, I could meet them.

"Sure," I said inwardly. What I had already witnessed was beyond my capacity for belief. How much more impossible and outrageous could the evening get?

The ceiling in our bedroom sloped upward to a loft nearly two-stories tall. Among the rafters I saw a diverse group of spiritual beings reveal themselves. They looked like luminous angels whose faces seemed not only kind and benevolent, but also educated and wise.

"May I introduce the Healing Council. Its members consist of Earth guardians, gemstone guardians, inner-world physicians, and others whose mission it is to introduce the Earth-world to Gemstone Therapy."

The doctor and a petite, fair-skinned, luminous woman who seemed to be in charge of the Healing Council engaged in a conversation that I could not hear. Finally, she nodded as though giving her consent, and the doctor nodded back.

He said to us, "If you want to learn more about the healing properties of gemstones, then you may contact the gemstone guardians directly. These are the inner-world beings responsible for the energies of the various crystals on the planet. They are equivalent to the devas of the plant kingdom and the guardian angels of humankind."

Eagerly David agreed.

The council members looked to me for my response. I had become overly saturated with all this new experience, and was nearly catatonic. I simply nodded.

"I shall arrange a meeting to introduce you," the doctor said.

He and David discussed some other things, which I don't remember, and then he left my body as swiftly and easily as he had come in. He made sure that I was able to return to my body fully and completely and then disappeared.

I told David about my experience with the Healing Council and recounted details of the healing that I had seen in his leg. As I did, the doubt crept in. While David seemed so comfortable with this unusual happening, so at ease with it, I needed to digest it. The experience sat like a lump in my stomach.

What had just happened? Was it real or imagined? I would have dismissed it entirely, except for one undisputable fact: David was now pain free.

3

AM I GOING CRAZY?

*T*he next morning I sat at the kitchen table and telephoned an old friend. I called only one person, because I didn't want anyone else to know about the channeling. I felt terribly guilty about it. Instinctively, I felt channeling was dangerous, and I believed it would be frowned upon by others on my spiritual path, as we valued spiritual freedom. By channeling another being, I was giving up my freedom—not to mention my own body and voice. I wanted to fit in and be accepted in my community. A fear of being ostracized made me feel doubly cautious.

What also bothered me was that I had seen things that normal people never see. What had I done to open the door to such an experience? I couldn't think of a single thing.

Maybe I was going crazy.

"Your experience was really far out," Bill said. To my dismay, he did not share my doubts. Instead, he asked me to consider how new and exciting this opportunity was. He knew my love of adventure and suggested I appeal to it to help me cope.

"But..."

"Do you really care what other people think?"

"Well, no, but..."

"You know what wrongness feels like. Does this feel wrong?"

"No. It's just so outside my comfort zone that I'm doubting my sanity and my identity. I'm not sure who I am anymore. It feels as though my whole world has turned upside down."

Bill suggested I pursue the path that life was providing until it started to feel wrong. Foremost, I should keep my compass accurate by being true to my daily spiritual exercises.

While this sounded reasonable, when I hung up the phone, I felt truly alone. I looked out our kitchen window at the untended garden. I felt equally ignored. Neither my husband nor my best friend heard and understood my conundrums.

For the rest of the day, I tried to let go my misgivings by doing housework and taking care of our two young daughters, Emily and Eleena. Fortunately, David's leg pain had not returned. When the girls were asleep for the night, I was folding laundry on the bed when David walked into the bedroom and suggested we contact the inner-world doctor again.

"I have a ton of chores yet to do."

"It will be okay."

"I don't think now is a good time." I moved a stack of towels into the closet.

"I'm already feeling his presence. I think I need a follow-up treatment, before the pain comes back."

I couldn't argue with that. "I'm still not sure that channeling is a good idea."

David folded some of the girls' clothes and put them in the basket. "But you are curious about the gemstones and their healing potential."

I couldn't argue that, either. After all, it was mostly gemstone energies that the doctor had used in David's healing session the night before. Their effects had been astounding.

Finally, my curiosity won and I acquiesced. I would do it one more time—just to make sure David's leg was okay.

When the laundry was done, we sat on the edge of the bed and went into a meditative state. We sang the word HU a few times, because it was a mantra we loved to sing, and doing so opened our hearts.

Soon I saw the brown-robed monk appear in my inner vision. "My husband would like to speak with you," I said.

At the same time, I felt the presence of a spiritual master and then saw him in my inner peripheral vision. His knee-length maroon robe and short black hair and beard identified him as Rebazar Tarz. He was a favorite inner teacher of mine, who works closely with my spiritual guide, Harold Klemp. Rebazar is a spiritual master beloved by many, who helps people regardless of their religious upbringing, if they ask.

As familiar as Rebazar was in books and artwork, I was not accustomed to seeing the inner master. I was not yet comfortable having my inner senses working so well.

"Is it okay to channel this being?" I asked Rebazar.

I awaited a warning or at least a bit of advice, but the master said nothing. Nor did his expression change. He simply sent me love. I took this as permission to have whatever experience I wanted and knew he would be there in case I needed him. Indeed, he stayed close while I gave the monk permission to enter my body.

To be sure my own thoughts did not interfere, I stepped out of myself once again and stood behind my shoulder. From this out-of-body viewpoint, our bedroom and its meager furnishings were brighter and lighter than their physical counterparts.

"You may call me 'Hahn,'" the doctor told us.

"Dr. Hahn?" David asked.

"We don't use titles where I come from. 'Hahn' will suffice."

Hahn asked permission to inspect David's leg, and then used my eyes to see inside of it. I was fortunate to be able to identify what I believe Hahn was looking at. First, I recognized layers of tissues, and identified muscle fibers, nerves, and vessels.

Then Hahn shifted his perspective and we saw the molecules and atoms that comprised these tissues, and the life energy that flowed through them. As though stepping back to see a wider perspective, we then examined the leg's emotional-body counter-part, then its causal or karmic layer, and also its mental essence. At each layer, unwanted or imbalanced energies were revealed. Hahn removed or harmonized them by pouring his precious liquids here and there.

I could now more clearly recognize the gemstone energies in these liquids and marveled at the instantaneous effect they had on the leg's energies. The body seemed to recognize the gemstone energies and readily accept them.

While Hahn outwardly conversed with David about his health concerns—using my voice to talk to him—inwardly he spoke to me about the gemstones. We were having a separate conversation. This dual consciousness seemed so natural while it was happening that I didn't question it. Hahn and I simply became engrossed in a conversation that was completely telepathic and our own.

"Are those liquids you are using actually colored, or am I seeing the light that emanates from them?"

The question seemed to amuse him. I thought I could hear him thinking, "Of all the things she could have asked about, she chose this."

"What do you sense?"

"I think I'm seeing the energies."

"You are correct. They are formulated using the color-ray-bearing gemstones. You'll find one for each color of the rainbow."

"Color-ray-bearing gems?"

"The gemstones whose mission it is to carry pure color frequencies on Earth."

"Why does the body respond to the gemstone energies so readily?"

"Earth provides gemstones because their energies help living things remain in balance. Herbs do the same thing, but their reach and approach is different. While herbs work mostly physically and somewhat energetically, gemstones work exclusively on the body's energies and its energetic counterparts. I'm sure you know that you are far more than your physical flesh."

Before I could agree, David asked a question that caught my attention. He wanted to know what type of doctor Hahn was and where he'd gotten his training.

"Gemstone Therapy is practiced commonly and openly in the inner worlds," Hahn replied. "We have clinics, hospitals, and universities devoted to the healing benefits of the mineral kingdom. I have studied this work for many years and have been appointed as an advisor to the healing council. I have also been asked to guide you in your work with the gemstones."

"When will we meet the gemstone guardians?" David asked.

"The assignment will be given formally sometime soon."

The assignment? Meeting the gemstone guardians meant I would once again see and hear things beyond the veil. I guessed I would be channeling them, too.

"Is it safe?" I asked Hahn.

"What are your concerns?"

I felt a swell of emotion come forward and forced back tears. We had two young daughters ages six and two. (I had yet to give birth to our son.) My children needed me, and I loved being a mom. What if something happened to me and I couldn't take care of them?

"Is there any possibility I could get locked out of my body and not be able to come back?"

"That is not possible. You are always protected."

"Will I lose my mind or my individuality?"

"Again, not possible."

The answers still did not resolve my uneasiness.

Hahn and David discussed which guardians we might be working with, in order for David to obtain therapeutic-quality samples of their gemstones. Having the gems' physical presence during the interviews showed respect and would help me connect with the guardians I would soon be channeling.

Hahn went through each of the strands we already had and showed us which ones were therapeutic-quality.

He explained, "While a casual user might find uplifting benefits from any quality of gemstone, the art and science of Gemstone Therapy requires that you use only the highest quality specimens."

He compared medicinal herbs to gems. "In herbal medicine, the healing compounds of a plant are extracted and the fibrous, nonessential portion is discarded. You use only the pure essence of the herb. With gemstone spheres, you have to separate out the ones with too many flaws and inclusions in a process called highgrading. Then you have a collection of therapeutic-quality gemstone spheres, which express the pure essence of the crystal and which are suitable for Gemstone Therapy."

"Is there anything else we can do to prepare?" David asked.

"Get a tape recorder so that the words you hear won't be lost." Hahn assured us we had everything else we needed.

When our meeting ended, Hahn left my body and simultaneously, I reentered it. My body felt especially good afterward. I felt lighter and brighter. Was it because of his presence? Or was it because I myself had been watching from a higher plane and perhaps carried some of its vibrations back with me?

I looked for Rebazar. There he was in the corner of my eye. His presence was comforting, yet I still questioned the rightness of the journey ahead.

4

MAKING FRIENDS WITH
THE GEMSTONES

*T*he good feeling I had after channeling Hahn did not last long. I wasn't sure how I felt about meeting the gemstone guardians. It meant I'd be doing more channeling, and the thought made me feel uneasy.

I went to check on my daughters, who shared a bedroom and slept together in a full-sized bed. I got in under the covers beside them and listened to their soft breathing. The moonlight streamed through the window, shining moonbeams on their faces and casting shadows on the far wall. Mentally, I took a photograph. I wanted to remember forever their sweet, peaceful expressions.

Their serenity contrasted with my angst. Why was I struggling so much with these experiences? After all, it wasn't as though visions were new to me. I recalled the first one I ever had, which occurred when I was young. My family and I were standing on the shore of one of the Great Lakes. Nested in the clouds over the horizon, I saw a huge castle with turreted rooftops.

My mother didn't see it.

I described it to her.

"It's just your imagination."

Oh?

Then why couldn't I also imagine other things I wished to see around the castle, like flying horses and Tinkerbell fairies? Try as I might, I could not conjure these images. So I knew what I was seeing was real.

"If you ever tell me about a special experience," I whispered to my girls in the darkness, "I promise I will listen. I will not discount what you say."

Another experience of my childhood came to mind. I remembered one night when I was too sick to sleep. I felt very alone. Suddenly a light filled my room and the dolls I had neatly lined up on the cedar chest got up and began to dance. I delighted in watching them circle and turn.

Were these the imaginings of a feverish child? I might have been so convinced had I not recognized years later a painting of the one who had orchestrated this magic. He is a spiritual master named Fubbi Quantz.

I do not remember having "imagined" anything else until the fall of 1971 when we were living in England. I was ten years old, and my grandmother had come to visit. We kept the house pitch black at night, and once, on the way to the bathroom, I saw an angel surrounded in blue light coming down the hall toward me.

I screamed.

Seconds later my grandmother held me in her arms.

"It must have been me who you saw. We were both heading for the bathroom at the same time."

"What about the blue light?"

"You were dreaming."

Why would I be frightened by such beauty? I knew better than to voice my question aloud.

In the months that followed, a hunger started gnawing at me that I couldn't identify or name. Nevertheless, I took down the large Children's Bible from our bookshelf and immersed myself in it. I read the entire book twice, cover to cover. When I found a passage that fed my Soul, I would reread it over and over again, drinking in the solace and inspiration it gave me.

Clearly there had been a connection between my experiences with the light and my hunger for religion.

I looked back at my sleeping daughters, and realized that one day I should tell them these stories. I had taught them to sing HU and wanted to give them a solid background in spirituality, yet every individual has a journey of her own. What would be theirs?

The turning point when my spiritual quest truly began occurred in 1972 when we were back in the United States. I was in seventh grade. One day, the entire student body was sent to the parking lot because of a bomb scare.

Just having come back from England, and having skipped sixth grade, I didn't know anyone. Boys were especially strange and scary creatures. Since I had just spent two years in an all-girls convent school, I'd had zero interactions with them.

Suddenly a tall Italian boy—one who was the object of much admiration from the girls in my grade—wrapped his arms around me. Stunned, I froze. After a few seconds he let go. I was mortified. What did this mean? Why did he do that? I had no girlfriends with whom I could discuss the situation, and certainly I could not tell my parents.

God would have to help me.

As soon as classes ended, I hurried to our nearby church. Anxiously I climbed the steps and tried the front door. It was locked.

"God, I need you now."

I tried the side doors. They were locked too. God was on the other side of those big thick oak doors and dreadfully out of reach.

25

I sat on the church steps and wept.

When a consoling feeling overcame me, I opened my eyes and saw an angel standing in front of me. She or he (I couldn't tell) was a translucent white being and surrounded by light, which I decided might have been wings. This time I was not afraid.

"If you cannot find God inside the church," the angel said, "then you should look for Him elsewhere."

My despair was replaced by hope. I visited other churches with new friends I'd made, and spent hours at the library reading books on religion. In 1975, my guitar teacher gave me a book called *In My Soul I Am Free* by Brad Steiger, and our guitar lessons morphed into discussions on spirituality.

It took me a year and a half to read the book. Once I did, I discovered that Chapter Five fed me spiritually, and I would read and re-read the pages, drinking in the sustenance that the words gave me. I couldn't get enough. I wanted to learn to travel out-of-body like Paul Twitchell did. I wanted to experience the worlds of Light and Sound that he described in his books. Now, finally, my spiritual search had a clear direction.

Other than these islands of spiritual fascination, my life proceeded somewhat normally for a teenager. I went to high school, did chores, worked part time, and got along with my two younger brothers. I became vegetarian, learned to crochet and make quilts, collected and dried wild flowers, drew and photographed birds, played my guitar, wrote poetry, and read a lot. I talked on the phone with girlfriends (this was long before cellphones existed), and had a respectable social life.

I realized I was blessed to have found a spiritual path at such a young age. Many people I knew searched for years before they found a teaching that felt like home. Maybe that was one reason I didn't want to do anything to compromise it.

I understood that those on a quest for true spirituality—as I considered myself to be—should not pursue psychic abilities, which could distract the seeker on the path to God. But what happens when you are suddenly gifted with clairvoyance, clairaudience, and a passport to the inner worlds, perhaps because of your love for God?

I realized that I wasn't upset about seeing Hahn or the Healing Council, or even the possibility of meeting the gemstone guardians. My angst boiled down to this: if the goal was to keep my attention on the purest and most sublime relationship with God possible for me now, why would I want to engage in psychic abilities that originated in planes far below the highest?

Decades later I would realize the difference. To pursue psychic talents in lieu of God is a misguided allocation of one's attention. If these talents develop naturally, however, then you must find a way to use them to serve others—while keeping your heart, mind, and soul devoted to your spirituality.

The girls stirred in their sleep. Their movement pulled me from my reverie and I realized I was thinking too hard. I asked my spiritual guide if I could get some answers in the dream state, and went to sleep.

The next morning I awoke with the realization that I had been struggling with myself, and it was time to stop. I lingered in bed trying to remember what dreams conveyed this knowledge. None came to mind. I just knew I had to be gentler on myself and more accepting of my circumstances.

Fine.

I would try to make friends with the gemstones.

I got up, went about my day, and wondered how I'd do that.

That afternoon I got an idea. The girls were busy playing, so I stole some time and went to our bedroom. I got out the box that housed our gemstone collection and placed it on the bed.

27

Since David and I had been in the jewelry business for a few years, I was already interested in gemstones. On occasion, in bookstores, I had leafed through books that described their healing effects. The accounts differed so much among sources that I never took what I read seriously. So, it was with a healthy dose of skepticism that I opened the box.

At once, the Sodalite called to me. Perhaps it was its dark blue color that caught my attention. I picked up a Sodalite necklace and inspected the white streaks that ran through the blue—a characteristic of this gemstone. I marveled how each sphere was entirely different from every other. As individual as snowflakes.

I laid down on the bed and instinctively held the gems to my chest. I closed my eyes. My body felt quiet. Then something began to move inside of me. It wasn't a physical movement, and not something I could pinpoint or describe very well. It left me feeling freer inside.

I moved the Sodalite away, and held it at arm's length. Something shifted inside my body once again.

Were the gems causing this?

I held the Sodalite close. Sure enough, the sensation returned.

I sat up and rummaged through the box to find another necklace. This time I chose Leopardskin Jasper. This gem has a tan background with black and brown features that form circles on the surface of the stones.

I held a strand of the Jasper to my chest. This time the sensation was completely different. It felt as though key centers of my body, within my throat, brain, and torso, were trying to move synchronously with each other.

This was really strange.

I put down the Leopardskin Jasper and picked up a handful of milky-pink Rose Quartz spheres.

"Okay, Rose Quartz, show me something more tangible."

I held the gems close.

Nothing.

I took a deep breath.

Still nothing.

My experiences with the Sodalite and Leopardskin Jasper must have been flukes, I decided. Or figments of my imagination. Perhaps I really wanted to feel something from them and made up the sensations I thought I'd felt.

Of course! What other explanation could there be? I was simply making it up.

Then I started to cry.

Out of the blue, a swell of emotion came up, and I couldn't stop the tears. I had no idea where this came from, or why I was crying. I didn't feel sad. Yet, obviously, my body had volumes of unaddressed grief to release.

Later I would learn that it takes Rose Quartz a little time to penetrate the body. Its energies had reached in and began pulling out emotions I had stored within myself for who-knows-how-long.

I wept until I heard David walking down the hallway toward the bedroom.

Quickly I put the gems away and hid in the bathroom to dry my eyes. I wasn't ready to accept my own experiences—let alone share them with anyone.

One thing was clear. These gemstones really did have the power to affect a person.

I now understood why it was important to speak with the gemstone guardians. We needed to hear about the properties and potential of the gemstones from the beings who knew them best. I promised myself that whenever the guardians were ready for an interview, I would be too.

I had needed time to drum up the courage to accept this assignment with the gemstone guardians. This is my nature. I often need to mull something over before I can accept it. This tendency stayed with me, even years later when I had a mysterious prophetic dream and learned the identity of the five-letter word beginning with "H."

5

A FIVE-LETTER WORD
BEGINNING WITH "H"

The ambulance brought me to the hospital around 5:00 a.m. I was given a small colorless room. Bob showed up a few minutes later with an armful of magazines on cars and audio equipment that he was planning to read on our flight to Minneapolis. I had nothing to do to pass the time and felt too restless to sleep.

"I can't get comfortable."

"Do you want another pillow?"

"No."

Bob found one anyway and helped me arrange them.

"It isn't working," I said.

"What isn't?"

"I didn't realize I had a bump on my head. When I fell, my head hit the sink."

"How badly does it hurt?"

"Not much, but you'd think they would have checked my head."

"I think there's a bigger picture here." Bob sat down and opened a magazine.

I stared at the ceiling for what seemed like hours before a doctor finally arrived. "You probably had a stomach bug," he said.

"So we can go home?" I asked.

"We're waiting for your bloodwork to come in."

An hour or so later, a different doctor visited. "I'm the cardiologist on call this evening. Your blood test results revealed you've had a heart episode. It might have been a mild heart attack."

He wanted to give me an angiogram to find out if I had clogged arteries.

"Could we schedule it after we return from Minneapolis?" I asked. Our flight would leave in about three hours. We could still make it.

"You're not going anywhere today."

When the doctor left, I tried to get up anyway. We had a plane to catch.

My efforts were fruitless. My body would not move. Never had I felt so little energy—not even after child-birth. I plopped back down.

"You can go if you want," I said to Bob.

"You mean to the seminar?" He looked up from his magazine.

"You don't have to be here."

"I'll stay with you to see this through."

"You don't have to."

"It's you and me, Babe."

It was?

While I was having my angiogram, Bob sat in the waiting room next door. Later he told me that he had done a spiritual exercise to try to find out what was going on. What really was the bigger picture? As soon as he asked the question, a song written by Neil Young came on the radio. Riding on the airwaves these words repeated: "Searching for a heart of gold."

Bob knew in that moment why I was there. At first, he attributed the premonition as a spiritual healing of my heart; later he would realize it meant far more than that.

Meanwhile, I was having another one of many new experiences. I'd never been in an operating room. Never knew how cold it was or how hard and narrow the operating table was. Nor had I ever needed to surrender to the medical profession. Being one who values natural healing methods, I felt wary of the procedure and was unable to relax.

I thought back to my experience in the Peaceful Place. The memories were comforting. How tangible the presence of my spiritual guide had been! Despite being in an operating room—I felt reassured that right now I was exactly where I was supposed to be. This was a new feeling too. Up until now, my life seemed punctuated by moves from one discomforting situation to another. One of the worst, I left my family and the gemstones so many years ago.

"Your arteries are squeaky clean," the doctor announced and ruled out a heart attack.

They decided to keep me in the hospital over the weekend for observation and release me on Monday. Bob had nowhere to go, so they allowed him to room with me. With no extra cots available, he and I shared my hospital bed. If you've ever stayed in a hospital, you know what the beds are like. Bob and I were accustomed to cuddling as we slept, so the arrangement worked for us.

That Sunday, Bob went for a long walk and came back with a gift.

"To cheer you up."

"No one has ever given me a box of chocolates before," I said and eagerly opened it. Just as I was about to pick out a truffle, I remembered another part of the terrible dream I'd had. Along with the warning to start thinking about changing my H_ _ _ _, came a challenge:

"You are not to eat chocolate for a year."

I loved chocolate.

I remembered in the dream arguing about the command. Did I really have to?

The directive was uncompromising. So, from some unknown reservoir of strength and conviction within me, I made the commitment to give up chocolate for one year. This wasn't the type of promise you make to yourself to stop a habit and then two days later go back to your well-worn ways. I'd done that before—more than once. This time, I would keep my word. Letting go of chocolate would be one of the hardest things I'd ever done. In the end, it would be almost three years before I ate the food again.

Now my problem was how to tell Bob. I didn't want to hurt his feelings. I thought about the spiritual master who had eaten a poisoned meal because it had been a gift and wondered if I should do the same.

No. I had to obey.

So I told Bob about the dream. Fortunately he understood and enjoyed the chocolate for me.

That part of the dream was one of protection. At the time, it was essential to stay away from caffeinated products. In my heart's weakened state, it might not have survived the stimulation.

Speaking of caffeine, a few hours before they were going to release me from the hospital on Monday morning, I was sitting on the edge of the hospital bed looking at *Better Homes and Gardens*. Out of the blue, the espresso-grande rush returned. Once again it felt as though my insides were shaking uncontrollably. Only this time, it was far less intense. I knew I could keep my composure by focusing intently on what I was reading.

In seconds, my room flooded with nurses, who all seemed very excited.

"Are you okay?"

"I'm fine."

"You're not fine," one of them said and made me go back to bed.

The heart monitor I was wearing had revealed ventricular tachycardia, also known as V.T., or v-tach. While it passed in about twenty seconds, now my doctors had evidence that my heart was, indeed, not fine. They transported me via ambulance to a nearby hospital that specialized in cardiac care.

There I learned that, in addition to v-tach, I also had cardiomyopathy, a disease of the heart muscle that manifests as an enlarged heart.

"V-tach is how people who otherwise seem perfectly healthy suddenly drop dead," a cardiologist told me. He rattled off a few names of athletes this had happened to. "In v-tach, the heart starts flopping like a fish newly caught and blood can't get to the brain or anywhere else."

He held my chart and tapped it rhythmically with his finger. "During your episode, did you check your pulse?"

"No."

"If you had, you may have found it speeding out of control, perhaps over two hundred beats per minute."

V-tach is a fatal type of arrhythmia. My doctors would call it near-fatal, because in fact, it hadn't killed me yet.

"It's a miracle you are still alive," the doctor said. He didn't believe me when I told him I'd endured the feeling for two long hours. Plus another ninety minutes after a short sleep. He thought I was exaggerating.

No wonder I felt so depleted. My body must have been using all its resources to stay alive.

To keep me alive, the doctor inserted an automated implantable cardioverter defibrillator (Bob and I called it an I.C.D.) into the left side of my chest, just under the skin beneath my collar-bone. It was a little smaller than a deck of cards. (I hear that these days they are even smaller.) If my heart started to beat wild-ly again, the I.C.D. would start pacing my heart rate out of the danger zone. If that didn't work, it would disperse an electrical current that would shock my heart back into a normal rhythm.

At least, that was the theory.

A few days later, just before they were about to send me home, I was struck once again with v-tach. My cardiologist and a flurry of nurses flew to my side and got busy.

The doctor explained that the arrhythmia was occurring at a lower heart rate than my I.C.D. was set to account for. Apparent-ly, my heart was able to flop like a fish even at a rate under 100 beats per minute. He promised to reset the device. In the mean-time we waited for an anesthesiologist to sedate me before he used the external defibrillator to make my heart beat properly again.

Meanwhile, I felt my energy level dropping. I began dipping into the Peaceful Place. The thick gray mist began to encroach, and I could feel myself slipping irretrievably toward the light on the horizon.

"Hurry up," I said.

"It will hurt. We're waiting for the anesthesiologist."

"Hurry up."

The doctor said some legalese to protect himself. He placed one paddle on the front of my chest, and another on the side. The electricity surged through me, and I shouted out.

Nothing changed.

Again they shocked my heart.

Again I shouted out.

My heartbeat returned to normal.

For the next several hours, I rested in a strange zone be-tween awake and asleep. The Peaceful Place was a breath away.

I heard Bob's voice, singing softly:

"You are my sunshine, my only sunshine.
You make me happy when skies are gray.
You'll never know dear, how much I love you."

Maybe I didn't know.

When I was awake enough to talk, we began to converse at a level of intimacy and enjoy a type of closeness that was new to us. At that time, I felt our relationship had an uncertain future, and yet, in those few hours, its true depth and potential began to reveal itself.

This was the first of many times when Bob would sing to me. Later on, occasionally—and only when I was really sick— he would add the final line.

"Please don't take my sunshine away."

I believe this was done unconsciously on his part, however, I was acutely aware of the sentiment. I really didn't think he loved me that much. Nonetheless, his presence felt deeply nourishing, and over the next few years, I began to rely on it.

The next time the doctor visited us, he told me that I had to take a certain drug to keep my heartrate under control. They could not let me leave the hospital until my body had a certain relatively high level of it, which could only be achieved intravenously. Thereafter, I could maintain this high level with oral doses. They didn't tell me that, intravenously, this drug destroys your veins. By the end of my twelve days in the hospital, both my forearms would be swollen twice their size, bright red, and bruised.

My dad flew in from Texas as soon as he heard of my heart condition. He would visit every time I had extended stays in the hospital. My brothers, both Lt. Colonels in the Air Force, also came. Paul drove up from Dover, Delaware, and Brian found a creative way to get leave from his station in

Afghanistan. John and Larrie, two family friends, also visited. My family's attendance was deeply meaningful beyond the small talk we enjoyed.

My heart failed, and everyone grew closer.

Every day Mom visited with Kellan, who always arrived with smiles and hugs. They were the best medicine I'd gotten yet. She would climb up onto my hospital bed and play with the buttons that adjusted the position of the mattress. We would cuddle, and she would show me the pictures she had made for me. Some of her drawings reflected sadness and fear—the emotions she was feeling, although unable to express. These were the pictures I didn't hang up on my bulletin board.

"When are we going home, Momma?"

"When I'm better."

"Tomorrow?"

"Soon. This is your special time with Grandma." I was unable to face my own emotions and had no clue how to help Kellan with hers.

One day, a cardiologist we had never seen before visited. He explained, in no uncertain terms, that my heart was very sick. Tests showed my heart was severely enlarged and had a very low ejection fraction. Ejection fraction is a measure of how strongly your blood is pumping through your body. My ejection fraction was around 10; normal is around 55.

In the months to come, I would see even lower numbers.

"With an ejection fraction of 10, you won't have the capacity to do very much. You won't be able to go back to work, and you won't be able to take care of your children."

"Why not? Exactly how long will it take for my heart to heal?"

He looked at me without answering. Then he said, "I suggest you get on the heart transplant list as soon as you get back home."

Bob and I were both speechless. I felt shocked by his words and kept silent so I would not have to choke on tears. Nevertheless, now I knew the identity of the five-letter word in my dream. It was time to start thinking about changing my H E A R T.

6

LIVING WITH HEART FAILURE

*I*t wasn't easy to accept the fact that I needed a new heart. When the doctor who told me I should get on the heart transplant list left my hospital room, Bob and I agreed it was inappropriate to hear such big news from a doctor we hadn't ever spoken to before.

Bob put his arms around me. "That doctor had no right to tell you that."

"I want a second opinion," I said. Secretly we hoped the diagnosis from another doctor would be different.

It wasn't.

After the second doctor left, I lowered the back of my bed so that I could lie flat, and pulled the covers over my head. I wanted to be somewhere else, just to think. Instead, my emotions took over. I felt a stream of them: shock, horror, anger, sadness, and disbelief. I also realized that hiding under the covers was ridiculous.

I pulled the sheet off abruptly, which startled Bob.

"What if they're wrong?"

He hesitated, and then said gently, "What if they're not?"

I turned my head away from him. Handling a diagnosis is a lonely journey.

41

I thought about others' experiences I'd heard or read about. Some people, upon hearing they have a terminal illness, resign to die. They've been beaten up enough this lifetime and are okay to let it all go.

Others rally hidden resources and take steps to get better. They take responsibility for their health through self-exploration and self-healing. They are willing to look carefully at the traumas and tragedies that may have spurred the imbalances that eventually led to their physical condition. They are brave and courageous souls, and they outlive their prognosis by many years.

Still others refuse to see beyond their physical condition. Despite the pain, it's easier to disregard limiting beliefs, negative attitudes, or toxic emotions that may be lurking beneath. They are certain their ailments are physical and don't bother to look within and heal possible causes.

What would be my path?

What the doctors said I needed was too big to grasp. Too far-fetched.

Heart transplant? No way.

I looked to my spiritual guide for help. I tried to imagine Harold's face—fair skin, short brown hair, high forehead, glasses. I often see him in my mind's eye wearing blue clothing.

This time, I saw nothing.

Maybe I was trying too hard.

I relaxed and sang HU inside my head. After a few minutes I had a feeling that no matter what, I would be okay. In fact, right there and right then I reminded myself that I was okay—whether the doctors' diagnosis was wrong or right.

At the very worst, I'd end up back in the Peaceful Place—and that wouldn't be so bad.

Twelve days after I had been admitted to the hospital, I was released. Bob suggested I move in with him so he could take care of me. We weren't ready for this step, but life gave us no choice.

This was when I started to ask myself why my heart failed? I didn't smoke or drink. I exercised, took vitamins, and ate organic foods. One friend suggested, "Maybe you were a Mayan priest in a past life. Maybe you cut out others' hearts—maybe your surgeon's. Now it's his turn to cut out yours."

I looked within, could find no affinity with the Maya, and said to myself no, that was not why.

The truth was, I wasn't ready to hear the answers. When they came years later, I would realize that the heart failure was a step I had to take before I could return to my gemstone journey.

Without the gemstones' assistance, I think I did pretty well at coping with my heart failure. You would too. It's only when you realize the type of energetic support gemstones can give you that you miss them when they're not there.

Back in the 1980s when I was working with the gemstones, I would sometimes leave my necklaces behind when we traveled—wondering if being without them really made a difference. I was such a skeptic. When my youngest brother got married, I took my three little children by myself, from Oregon, where we lived, to Tucson, where the wedding took place. It was also a family reunion. I chose not to wear my gemstones because I didn't feel brave enough to explain them to my relatives.

After being accustomed to the support the gems provided, I felt vulnerable and awkward. I managed, although I would have done so much better with them. Their energies would have given me extra strength and stamina to travel with the kids, emotional strength to deal with the undercurrents between family members, who had recently divorced, and I probably wouldn't have felt so travel-weary when I got home.

Then, as now, my journey would have been easier had I worn the gemstone necklaces.

To support myself after the heart failure, I would have chosen some of the basic ones simply because my health was so out of balance. Among my first choices would have been Quartz. Today, I pair Frosted Quartz with Clear Quartz of optical quality, to promote harmony and balance, and thus invite a full complement of healing energies into the body.

Two or three times a day, I would have placed across my body a collection of five necklaces I call the Foundation Five. These are particularly grounding and nourishing and meet the body's needs for energetic balance in a variety of ways. Foremost, they help balance the five phases of the life-cycle, which have been identified as the five elements: water, wood, fire, earth, and metal.

Certainly, I would have also tested which color ray I was most deficient in and worn the gems that carried that ray.

I would also have been wearing Morganite, whose energies are like vitamins for the emotional body. I pair it with White Beryl, which purifies, and Rhodonite, whose energies are emotionally grounding and support courage. A well-nourished emotional body is less likely to feel numb and despondent and is more capable of being in touch with its true feelings. At this point in my journey, it would have been helpful to be clearer about how I really felt.

I cannot say that had I worked with such and such a gemstone that I might have avoided certain experiences. That's not what Gemstone Therapy is about. The gemstone energies smooth the sharp, rough edges of an experience or they help us be more aware of what's really going on. They don't take the experiences away.

In addition, I have found that gemstone necklaces are good at balancing energies throughout my body and being. When I feel more balanced, it's easier to handle uncomfortable situations. It's easier to digest bad news. I feel more like myself and am able to respond to situations more gracefully and intelligently.

I certainly could have used a little more grace at my first appointment with a local electrophysiologist, a cardiologist who specializes in the electrical malfunctioning of the heart. In other words, he took care of patients with v-tach, like me. During a brief visit, the doctor told me with the utmost nonchalance that he was going to replace the I.C.D. unit they'd given me in the previous hospital with a "better" one.

In a daze, I walked out of his office with Bob and into the hallway. We started to the elevator. I was feeling increasingly uncomfortable about the situation. Why did I need another surgery? What was wrong with the I.C.D. I already had? Then my feet froze—they wouldn't let me go farther.

"Bob, I need to go back."

For the first time since my heart failure, my emotions surged to the surface. They fueled me with the gumption to storm into the receptionist's office and ask where the doctor was.

She was deceptively vague, so I barged into his office. Fortunately he was alone, sitting behind his massive desk, which was covered with paperwork.

If he was surprised to see me, he didn't show it.

I was polite, yet firm. "I'm sorry to disturb you, but I need to know what is going on. Out of the blue something happened to my heart. Two weeks ago, I was doing karate, now I can hardly walk. I just received a new I.C.D. at a top cardiology hospital, from one of the best cardiologists in the country, and now you're telling me this unit isn't good enough?"

By now I was in tears.

The doctor listened stoically. "Your heart has probably been sick for a long time," he said in a measured tone. "It reached a point where it could no longer continue to function normally, and then it failed."

"Why do I need a new I.C.D.?"

"We use a different medical-devices company. Our comput-ers don't talk to the unit that you were given at the other hospi-tal. I'm sure it's a fine unit. You are welcome to continue your care at the hospital where you received it. If you want your care here, you need a unit I can work with."

"This is all very new and unexpected."

"Changing an I.C.D. is quick. You'll be asleep, so it's pain free. Call when you want an appointment."

I cried for a long time after we left his office.

Once all the tears were out, it was time to be brave again, to face whatever was ahead with as much neutrality and acceptance as I could. There was no way we were going to commute to the other hospital four hours away. I would have to get the I.C.D. replaced. I vowed to greet my fate with a joyful heart. No matter how sick my physical heart might be, my spiritual one was going to shine.

On New Year's Eve, 2002, we attended a party at a friend's fitness club. By this time I was looking better and feeling well enough to take frequent trips to the potluck table.

In case someone asked what had happened to me, I tried to think of funny answers but was coming up empty-handed. The humor came unexpectedly. I was talking with someone who heard I had been in the hospital. I thought she knew why.

"Do you want to see the implant?" I asked her. I moved the collar of my shirt to one side to reveal the I.C.D. sticking out beneath my collarbone.

Her face instantly reddened and she threw her arms up to cover her eyes.

When I had mentioned "implant," she thought I had gone into the hospital for breast implants. The laughter that ensued was healing and heart-warming.

Now I knew that Bob was right. The five-letter word beginning with H also referred to humor. I needed to take life less seriously.

At the end of January 2003, we moved out of Bob's apartment and into my house. I found it harder to keep my humor as I began to feel progressively sicker. One afternoon, I was sitting at the kitchen table and suddenly had no more energy to do anything—not even to go back to bed. I folded my arms on the table and rested my head on them. I promised myself I'd hang on until Bob got home from work. He would be able to assess the seriousness of my symptoms.

As I waited, I drifted into the Peaceful Place. I rested as though suspended in the gray mist and I cannot say how much time passed.

It may have been hours before Bob and his son, Ryan, found me. It was time for another ambulance ride to the emergency room. I'd already gone there once from his apartment.

"Do you have health insurance?" is the first question the hospital admitting staff asks.

Being sick requires that you are somewhat prepared financially. After two divorces, I did not have any financial cushion to fall back on. I had zero savings and not much in my checking account. However, I did have health insurance...all because of Kellan and the blessings of inner guidance.

The year prior to my heart failure, Kellan was attending a daycare center that was landscaped with a retaining wall. The wall was about a foot wide and began at ground level. Along the path to the parking lot, the wall grew taller to hold back a small hillside. At the entrance to the parking lot, the wall was shoulder height.

When I picked up Kellan at the end of the day, she would pull away from me—no matter how firmly I held her hand— and hop onto the retaining wall.

"Kellan, hold my hand!"

She ignored me.

Nothing I could say or do would stop her from running the length of the wall and hopping down onto the grass by the parking lot. Although I feel I'm an easy-going parent, I believe I am relatively strict when it comes to my children's safety. In this instance, I had absolutely no control. Why was this child so persistent?

"Buy health insurance," said a strong nudge. It made sense. In case Kellan fell—and at worse suffered a broken arm—I might be set back financially, but not ruined. The problem was, I learned I could not purchase insurance just for my daughter. I had to buy the policy for me and add her onto it. So I did. The policy had a six-month probation period during which the insurance company would not pay for anything.

The seventh month after I purchased the insurance, my heart failed.

When the hospital staff asks if you have health insurance and you say "yes," they make some phone calls to find out what kind. Maybe it shouldn't work like this; however I'm convinced that without the comprehensive health insurance that I had, I would not have been given the high degree of care that I received. And without a new heart, I would not be alive today.

By the spring of 2003, my heart health continued to decline, and I lived most of the time in bed. My quality of life was dictated by my blood pressure. For me, normal was 90 over 60. What a blessing it was to be there. I could stand upright, walk, talk, read, write, think, and watch television if I wanted. At times, my blood pressure would reach other levels, each of which was a world of its own.

At 80 over 50, I would feel more weakened than usual, although I could still eat, read, and watch T.V. Still, I would have to limit my activity. I'd calculate my every move and then decide if the energy expended and the tiredness I'd feel afterward was worth it.

At 70 over 40, I would call Bob at work to let him know my blood pressure was dropping, and I might need him home. In the world of 70 over 40, I could not do much besides lie in bed and look at the elephants printed on the wallpaper. Even watching television took too much effort. I couldn't think or hold a conversation. The rows of elephants marching among golden leaves were my best entertainment.

When the pressure dropped to the other-worldly 50 over 30, it took all my strength and Bob's coaching just to keep breathing. Every inhale and every exhale took conscious effort. When this became too hard to maintain, we would call 911, and I'd spend the night in the emergency room.

Once I dropped into 50 over 30 when my friend Larry came to visit. I always hoped I'd be at least in the 80 over 50 world when I had visitors. I had so few of them, it was always a joy to have someone new to talk to. Graciously, Larry lay down on the bed facing me, taking each breath with me, coaching me until Bob got home and took over.

If I had been working with gemstones at this point, there's no doubt in my mind I would have been holding a necklace during the blood pressure drops. Not only for the grounding energy it provides, which can feel strengthening, but also for solace. There's something intrinsically comforting about wearing a piece of the Earth around your neck or as a bracelet—or clutching it against your chest during a crisis.

At 90 over 60, or even 80 over 50, I had enough energy to handle visits from only one of my two youngest daughters at a time. I taught them each to dial 911, just in case, and also how to phone Bob.

This came in handy once when AriaRay was visiting. She was about seven years old at the time. After giving her a bath and brushing our teeth together, I could feel my blood pressure dropping. Then my heart started to beat weirdly.

I lay down on the bathroom floor.

"Aria, do you remember how to call Bob?"

She answered by hopping up to get the phone. Proudly she dialed his number. Then she sat beside me, chatting about this and that to keep me company until he came home.

After that episode, my cardiologist decided to try a special type of I.C.D. that had an extra wire to stimulate a second portion of my heart. He expected this might normalize my heart rhythms, which sounded more like a galloping horse rather than a steady and healthy da-dum, da-dum.

He also suggested a variety of tests and experiments. In one, I lay on my back under an x-ray machine with dye in my veins while I rode a recumbent bicycle. It was the most ridiculous thing they ever made me do. Meanwhile, a cadre of medical personnel watched a television monitor that showed how the dye was flowing through my heart.

The results were definitive. My heart had expanded in size so much that two valves were unable to close. With exercise, the blood actually flowed backwards! No wonder I felt well only when I remained motionless.

It was time to think seriously about changing my heart.

7
MEETING THE GEMSTONE GUARDIANS

$\mathcal{M}$ost of the time when I do a spiritual exercise and look within, nothing happens. I sit on my couch looking for the light and chanting HU or another mantra, and I stare at a blank screen. On special occasions, a veil parts and the inner worlds welcome me with their splendor. This is what happened that night in 1987 when we were formally given the assignment to work with the gemstone guardians.

We sat on a couch that we had moved into the bedroom. It would be a special place to sit when we did the upcoming interviews.

Hahn appeared moments after I closed my eyes. I wasn't expecting him.

"Let's go. They're waiting for you."

While my physical body sat in our bedroom, my spiritual-self stood up and followed Hahn right through the walls of our house and into the night sky. It felt as though we were a hundred feet above the ground, although all I could see was a light gray mist and the back of Hahn's head.

We stood upright as we flew and I sensed we headed east. I heard a sound like rustling leaves and felt air moving against my skin. In time, the sound of the wind grew louder. Soon enough

I noticed we were moving over a mountain range. It was daylight wherever we were and I could see the land below. One snow-capped peak after another glistened in the morning sunlight as we passed overhead.

We slowed and descended into a valley where a group of people mingled around a large crystal, twice the height of the average man. The crystal reflected light that pulsed in a compli-cated rhythm, as though it was taking part in a conversation.

I wanted to land closer to the crystal, but Hahn directed us to set down near the edge of the gathering. My feet touched the ground, which was bare and somewhat rocky. The snowline began in the nearby foothills and the white-capped mountains surrounded us.

It was so beautiful here! The air was crisp and fresh, and although my mind suggested I should feel cold, I wasn't.

"Welcome friends!" said a wizardly man, whose purple eyes immediately caught my attention. He wore a long white beard and a hooded white robe, and I was sure his skin had a hint of purple in it too.

"The Guardian of Amethyst," Hahn announced.

He spread his arms to greet me and David, who I saw stand-ing with us.

"Thank you," I said.

I could sense the specialness of the occasion and guessed the people in this gathering were the gemstone guardians. The Am-ethyst Guardian confirmed their identity. He explained that they were discussing a book that would soon be written about them. It would contain a series of interviews that they would give.

I knew David and I would be giving those interviews, al-though I hadn't expected they'd be compiled into a book. Of course. The idea made perfect sense. It was time that people knew the truth about gemstones and their energetic value. Who better to tell the tale then the gemstone guardians themselves?

What better way to share the information than in a book?

The assembly was informal. The guardians mingled as any group would at a party.

The Guardians of Ruby and Carnelian approached me. They're both female. The Ruby Guardian looked about sixty, and the Carnelian Guardian looked to be in her mid-thirties. Their beauty and vitality were enviable. They shared an air of personal power as well as the self-discipline to contain it.

"Welcome," the Ruby Guardian said. She was taller than her companion and wore a straight floor-length red gown embedded with rubies. "I've been looking forward to meeting you again."

Had we met before? I wracked my memory.

"It was lifetimes ago."

"The Guardian of Ruby is the oldest among us," the Guardian of Carnelian explained. "She tends to see everything in the moment. This is one of her abilities. The passage of time does not dilute Ruby's energies, all that Ruby ever has been or known is accessible right now."

Ruby had always seemed like a powerful gemstone. Now I knew why.

The Guardian of Carnelian's dress caught my attention. Her floor-length gown consisted of multiple layers of sheer, glistening orange fabric, and artfully embellished with carnelian beads. I wished I could see what her shoes looked like.

The Guardian of Carnelian swirled, and in doing so her dress lifted slightly.

Oh, right—thoughts are heard here. Her shoes were carved of Carnelian.

This guardian seemed more amicable and relaxed than the Ruby Guardian. I felt as though we could be friends. Her skin had an orange tone that looked most unusual. I assumed this was carnelian energy rubbing off on her.

53

"We have so much to share with you," she said. "We're all very excited to get started."

"In time, the interviews have already occurred," the Guardian of Ruby said in her business-like tone. "Everything you're about to do has already been done. This viewpoint will be a key to your success in this project."

The Guardian of Carnelian chimed in. "I can't wait to share information about the color rays. People need to know how life energy actually nourishes the body, and how they can use gemstones to work with the color rays directly."

I wanted to hear more about the color rays, and sensed that I would, in time.

What the Ruby Guardian said answered my question about having known her before. Indeed we had met. My present incarnation was an opportunity to complete an assignment that I'd started long ago. I'd read how people had used and misused crystals during the age of Atlantis. I sensed something had not gone well in a lifetime I'd had at that time, and here was my chance to make amends.

A deep horn blew in the distance and echoed through the valley. It summoned everyone to the circle around the central crystal.

As I walked forward, I noticed every guardian looked unique, as though each had come from a different country and was wearing his or her native costume. Hahn would probably tell me I was also seeing their individualized energies.

When everyone was gathered, I expected someone would step forward to address us. Instead, the guardians closed their eyes. Well, most of them did. I noticed some chose to keep them open and just relax their gaze. That was my choice, too. I didn't want to miss anything.

My attention was drawn to the crystal in the center of our

circle. Somehow I knew—although maybe I'd picked up someone's thoughts—that the Earth herself was about to speak to us
through this crystal. Apparently, the Earth had consciousness,
intelligence, and individuality, and somehow she could communicate with us.

The Earth's first message came as a feeling. I felt a wave of
gratitude flood through me. I also witnessed a genuine return
wave of gratitude that erupted from within me for the Earth, for
everyone present, and for this entire experience. It came sponta-
neously and gave me another hint that my connection with the
gemstones reached far beyond what my human awareness was
presently capable of.

The next message the crystal sent involved the grand
connectivity among all things. This too came through as a
feeling. I could clearly feel how everything in the universe,
no matter how large or small, is connected by the life-energy
that manifested it and that continues to enliven it. I could
feel how all are healed and moved and allowed to grow and
unfold by this same energy.

Suddenly, I could see the relationship between every individual here and every star, planet, living being, molecule, and
atom, like a network of tiny golden threads. I was flooded with
gratitude for the connectivity among all life and the sense of
oneness it inspired. Moreover, the Earth was vitally connected
to everyone here. These were the guardians of her crystals, and
David and I were the ones charged with telling their story.

Something shifted in the circle and everyone began opening his
and her eyes. Conversations resumed. I wondered if each individual
had heard the same communication. No, each had heard his own.

Another woman in the circle caught my attention. I remembered her as the head of the Healing Council that we had met
previously.

The Guardian of Amethyst introduced us. "The Guardian of Diamond."

"The Diamond Guardian?" I felt awed.

"She is also the overseer of the gemstone guardians."

A petite woman stepped toward us, smiling broadly. Her hair was light brown, long and wavy, and sparkled in the sunlight as though it was adorned with diamonds. She had a spring in her step and her aura exuded joy. Pinpoints of white light and flashes of all seven colors of the rainbow flashed on and off around her.

She also seemed very familiar, and I wondered if I'd worked with her too in the past, perhaps when I knew the Ruby Guardian? I wanted to have a conversation with her, and hoped for an opportunity.

She formally addressed everyone and spoke about our assignment. Then to David and me she suggested that during our upcoming interviews I should speak my experiences into a tape recorder and that David should ask questions. As though responding to my unvoiced concern, she assured me I would be safe. Her final advice was to write with love, light, and enjoyment.

When it was time to leave, Hahn escorted us back home. My concerns about the interviews had evaporated, and I eagerly looked forward to learning more about the healing capabilities of gemstones.

A few weeks later, we had our first meeting with the Guardian of Quartz. David and I brought out some strands of Quartz spheres and had a tape recorder ready. We closed our eyes and relaxed.

Within moments, my inner vision opened to a scene of the stereotypical heaven. Billowy white clouds surrounded us. I guessed this was a location that my mind would find comforting so that it wouldn't object to some of the new experiences I was about to have. The last thing I needed now was to self-doubt or become fearful. Thankfully, the ground felt solid beneath my feet.

The Guardian of Quartz was tall, dressed in a white cape that covered a white linen shirt and pants. His straight hair was blond and cut short in the front, longer on the sides, and shoulder length in back. It was symmetrical, like a crystalline matrix.

He greeted us warmly and held out a single quartz crystal point in his hands. It transformed into a cluster, and then the cluster morphed into a single large quartz sphere. I took that as an invitation and looked into his brown eyes. As he gazed back into mine, I thought for a moment that I'd be lost in the light that surrounded him.

Instead, I was drawn into his aura. Instinctively, I turned to face the direction he was looking, and suddenly I could see what he saw. I could also feel what was in his heart and could speak with my physical voice the words he wanted to share.

Meanwhile, my body sat quietly on the sofa in our bedroom. It was late at night and because the children usually slept deeply, I didn't worry about being disturbed.

I found that channeling the gemstone guardians was not so bad after all. In fact, the experience was exhilarating. Harold, my spiritual master, or Rebazar, was always in my peripheral vision, which gave me a great deal of reassurance. I always felt stronger and healthier after being immersed in a gemstone's energies, though the channeling would eventually take its toll.

Over the next several months, I channeled each of thirty different gemstone guardians. I spoke my experiences into a tape recorder and David steered the interview with questions. During the day, I would transcribe the recordings. I worked with a brilliant wordsmith, Elizabeth Barile, who taught me how to convert my verbal ramblings into concise writing and who did much of the editing herself.

The guardians supported what scientists and popular authors were, back in the 1980s, beginning to acknowledge: Matter and energy are interchangeable. This fact has a profound implication for health and health-improvement because we are not just physical beings. In fact, we are mostly energy. This energy permeates and surrounds us.

Our energy field recognizes gemstone energies and responds remarkably well to them. And why not? The Earth provides air, food, and water to keep us alive. She provides herbs to heal our bodies, and she provides minerals, in the form of crystals, to heal our energies. I believe our compatibility with gemstones also involves their simple atomic nature. Most gems are comprised of only a few different types of elements. The simplicity allows their healing energies to be instantly recognized and easily received.

The gemstone guardians taught us that gemstone spheres were specifically meant for healing, while gems in their raw form served the planet's needs. Crystals move energies linearly: in one end and out the other. A sphere's energies radiate evenly in all directions. When strung into necklaces and worn, their energies fill the body as well as the aura, to directly benefit the emotions, memory, and mind.

Spheres could be cut in such a way that they isolated the purest portion of the crystal, thus capturing its true essence. This was essential for a gemstone's energies to radiate unimpeded. It also gave the body an accurate sense of the gemstone's potential.

The guardians' message to those who wanted greater health was a dual approach. Go to health-care professionals as necessary. Take care of your body. But also take care of your energy field. Both approaches together would support health the best.

How do you take care of your energy field? Use healing gemstone spheres.

They can be worn all day or put in bed at night. While you are busy with your workaday world or your dreamtime, the gemstone energies smooth disrupted energies, clear blockages, nourish depletions, and resolve imbalances.

The guardians told us that healing gems would prove essential to ensure the health and survival of humankind. They hinted that the future promised assaults of an energetic, electromagnetic nature from many sources, most of which were, in 1987, still unknown. Healing gemstones would provide a solution for protection and, more importantly, adaptation to a new environment.

Thus began my work with healing gemstone spheres. I developed necklace designs with the help of the diamond guardian, wrote a home study course, and taught rudimentary treatment procedures. David took charge of building and running the administrative side of the business.

In early 1989 our son was born and, soon after, our book was published. Something seemed to change then. Suddenly people wanted to talk to us, editors wanted interviews, and our customers wanted workshops on how to work with the gemstones.

It was word-of-mouth that spread the gemstone guardians' message. People who grew up collecting rocks, who loved gemstones, who inherently knew that gemstones had healing powers...these were the ones who were attracted to our work and who were grateful to us for sharing it.

We got so much positive feedback that it inspired me to learn more. We had been told that enough information existed about each individual gemstone to fill an entire book, and I was excited to learn it all. I also enjoyed teaching.

On the other hand, talking publicly and giving interviews was clearly something I did not want to do. Finally, I felt the wrongness that my friend Bill had suggested I look out for. Every time I thought about it, I felt a brick wall in front of me, preventing me from moving forward.

"We need to promote the book," David insisted.

"I can't do it."

The inner guidance was very clear. Going public was something I could not do. I blamed it on my shyness and ineptitude; in reality, it just wasn't time. We hired someone else to do publicity for us with mediocre results.

A few short years later, in 1992, it became painfully apparent that I wasn't ready. Before I could share the work publicly and with passion, I needed to make some changes within myself.

Today, Gemstone Therapy is a sophisticated modality. To be capable of sharing the advanced methods—many of which Hahn had originally used on David's leg—required much more life experience. Foremost, I would have to separate my true feelings from the effects of the fears, ignorance, and intolerance of others. I would have to let go grief and resentment and open my heart to greater love. I would have to learn to stop doubting myself and fully accept my gifts as blessings. I would have to find my inner courage.

From the viewpoint of the outside world, I abruptly left. The lack of rightness that I sensed at the very beginning had never fully resolved. In fact, it smoldered and festered until I could not continue the work anymore.

I needed a change of heart, and I was going to get one, quite literally.

8

THE HEALING TEMPLE

*T*he first step to heart transplant is to win the approval of the transplant nurse. If you are successful, you can then be approved for transplant evaluation, which involves three days in the hospital for comprehensive testing.

Bob, Dad, and I attended the interview, which took place in a hospital meeting room. We sat at the end of a conference table designed for two dozen people. My support team occupied a discomfortingly small portion of the spacious room.

The nurse began with an overview of what was involved if I got on the list. I would carry a beeper and have a small suitcase ready. When I was called, I'd have to go to the hospital immediately—no matter where I was or what I was doing. If I got sick, I would be temporarily removed from the list.

Finally she said, "You need to be emotionally prepared to wait. In fact, the call for a new heart might not come in time."

Silence hung in the air while we digested this. My dad put a hand on my shoulder.

"What about the donor?" I asked.

"Most potential donors are victims of severe head trauma, brain aneurysm, or stroke," she explained. "They must be officially brain dead before donation is considered."

"Do you mean comatose?"

"Coma is not brain death. Brain death means the brain has zero activity and the patient cannot breathe without assistance. A physician must perform a series of tests to confirm brain death. Brain death is death." She pulled a pamphlet from her briefcase about organ donation.

"What about the family? Do they have a say in the donation?" Bob asked.

"Anyone who is a potential donor would have already consented to the gift. Either they enrolled in their state's donor registry when they obtained or renewed their driver's license, or by informing their family of their wishes."

"What if a person who has not enrolled becomes brain dead?" I asked.

"Then a representative of the Organ Procurement Organization will seek consent from the next of kin."

"If they give that consent?"

"The individual will be examined to see if he or she is suitable to serve as a donor. If it looks good, someone will contact the Organ Procurement and Transplantation Network to begin the search for matching recipients." She added, "Some of the tests you get during transplant evaluation will help them match you to a donor."

At the end of our meeting, the nurse looked at me thoughtfully. "I don't think you are a good candidate for heart transplant."

Her comment caught me off guard.

"Why not?" I whispered, my throat suddenly tight with emotion.

"Heart transplant is a big deal and you have only two people on your support team. Usually, this room is filled with family and friends who are committed to helping the patient through the long and arduous process. Not only will you need support before the transplant, but afterward as well."

"We are all one-hundred percent committed," my dad said.
"We are all she needs," Bob added.

Although my team was small, it was the best.

Then she looked at me and asked, "Do you really want a heart transplant?"

I looked at her blankly. At this point, I wasn't sure.

The nurse continued, "Afterward, you may feel as though you belong to the medical community. For the rest of your life you will take immuno-suppressant drugs, get regular testing and heart biopsies, and require frequent visits to a variety of different doctors."

She leaned forward, "Can you accept that, considering how much you also believe in natural living?"

She paused. "Don't answer now. Think about it."

Indeed, I thought about it. I was like a dog with a bone. On the one hand, I would get my life back. On the other, someone destined to die would, upon their death, bequeath me an organ. A part of this person would live inside me and, in a way, we would keep each other alive. Was I okay with that?

That night as I lay in bed, I wrestled with my thoughts and more concerns popped up. I wondered if it really mattered if I fought to retain the body I was given in this lifetime. Would it be better to fulfill my destiny in a different lifetime, with perhaps a healthier body? Was my heart transplant predestined? How much of a choice did I really have?

Finally, I was able to relax. When I crossed the threshold of sleep, I realized I had remained awake. I was lucid dreaming! This was a rare and treasured occurrence. I focused on details in the world around me so that I'd stay focused. I didn't want to crash back into my body and end the experience.

I was walking along a well-manicured path in a meadow filled with wildflowers. Bees and butterflies flitted about, and birds were singing. The meadow covered rolling hills that stretched for miles under the bluest sky. I suspected this was the supra-physical plane. This is a level of reality very much like Earth, only greener, bluer, and more beautiful. You might say it exists at a slightly higher vibration than the physical plane.

Someone who seemed familiar, but whom I didn't recognize appeared at my side, and then someone else, and then a group of us were walking together. The mood was happy and expectant.

After a while I saw in the distance a white building that reminded me of a Roman temple. I was glad we were walking toward it, as I was curious why this place also felt so familiar. When we got closer, I saw more clearly the white marble pillars and the long set of marble stairs leading up to the double front doors.

The road to the temple was lined with people, eager for something. A parade perhaps?

I slipped in behind the crowd, content to watch from the rear.

Then my entourage coaxed me onto the road. We walked toward the temple, and up the marble steps. When I reached the top and turned to look out at everyone, the crowd applauded with gratitude.

They had been waiting for me.

Then I understood. This was a healing temple and teaching facility that I would help to build—if I lived to build it. If I did not want a heart transplant, it would never come to be. In the next instant, I saw what would happen: the field where the temple was to be built was empty except for wild grasses.

I hadn't a clue why I would be building a healing temple. My return to the gemstone journey was still to come and not yet even a thought in the back of my mind. Nonetheless, if building a healing temple was my destiny, could I accept it? If so, where would I find the courage, or the resources, to manifest it?

Apparently, my heart transplant was not predestined. At every point along the way I had the choice to say, "This is not my path." While I felt the transplant was a choice that was mine to make, I was not going to be stupid about it. If a door opened that felt like an opportunity, I promised myself I'd step through it.

That door presented itself a week later.

I believe your entire life can change in one phone call. When the transplant nurse called, it did. I was sitting in my home office when the phone rang.

"You've been approved for heart transplant evaluation," she said, and gave me the phone number to call to make the appointment.

I felt surprised, elated, relieved, scared, and very grateful. In that moment I knew for certain: I wanted to be on the heart transplant waiting list.

That November, 2003, Bob brought me to the hospital for testing. To be eligible for heart transplant, they needed to be sure that I was healthy enough to survive the trauma of the surgery. Plus, because those who need a heart far outnumber the hearts that become available each year, they don't want to waste a good heart on someone soon to die of another failing organ.

Heart transplant evaluation would be the biggest examination of my life. For three days I would have to prove that I was worthy to receive the gift of life. My body, organs, and cells were all going to be tested to find out if they, we, I, deserved a second chance.

We needed to pass this test.

If we failed… well, the thought of living out my life in my present circumstances had become utterly unthinkable. I could not entertain a single thought about that possibility.

The blood tests came first. Refusing to faint after seeing the number of vials they had to fill was a test in itself. Then I was

65

admitted and given a room, which would be my home for the next three days. During that time, the medical staff evaluated my every organ and function. I received a breathing test, muscle strength test, and bone density test, plus ultrasounds, various types of scans, and mental and emotional evaluations.

After a respiratory system evaluation, I was wheeled into a waiting room, where again I experienced 50 over 30. I slumped in my wheelchair, without enough strength to call for help. I watched patients come and go, and the hands on the clock move steadily forward for minutes and then hours. I felt safe. I knew someone would come looking for me sooner or later, and finally someone did. My nurses were horrified that I'd been "lost." I found it amusing.

This experience, which I thought so hilarious, was a high point because the tests took their toll on me emotionally. At one point, while I was awaiting the next test, I remembered my childhood when I was always having stomach aches. I was accused of faking my symptoms just to get attention. Was that happening now?

"Bob, it's time to leave."

I'd had enough of this nonsense and got out of bed.

"Not now, Isa, the doctor's here."

"I've been faking my symptoms," I said to the doctor. "I'm really sorry for troubling you. I just wanted attention."

I noticed the doctor suppress a smile. His expression almost made me laugh too.

"You are not faking it." He waved my file. "I have the test results to prove it."

Denial was like an aspirin that took away a headache—for a little while. My body was not going to let me deny anything.

After all the tests were done, it took another couple of weeks for the results. When Bob and I visited my cardiologist, we felt upbeat and hopeful that I had passed them.

"I have good news for you," the doctor said, "and better news."

We couldn't wait to hear.

"You're a good candidate for transplant. But we think your heart problem may be corrected with open-heart surgery instead."

He explained that they wanted to try fixing my leaky valves first. During the procedure, the surgeon would also remove any patches of scar tissue that were burdening my heart. If the procedure worked, I could avoid heart transplant entirely.

I knew this was not my destiny and would be a waste of time and energy. Yet it was the next logical step and I had to take it.

So we went to visit the surgeon who would perform the operation. During our interview, I had the distinct impression he was looking at my internal anatomy. I'd never had such an experience before. Some men will look at your chest—this one was looking inside it. I can only guess he was considering what my heart looked like and what he might find when he got face to face with it. I considered it an odd way to look at a patient; I share it as a compliment to him and a testament to his proficiency. It made me feel confident that I was in good hands.

The surgeon looked at his calendar. "I can schedule you for January 22, 2004."

"That's my birthday!"

My exclamation surprised him.

"Yours will be a special gift," I explained.

He looked at me, perplexed. Perhaps he was seeing my face for the first time.

I looked forward to the surgery with a happy attitude, even to the point of being unable to sleep the night before because I felt like a child on Christmas Eve knowing Santa Claus was about to arrive for real.

I believed I would be getting my life back. I would never see 50 over 30 again.

*   *   *

"I have good news and bad news," the surgeon said when I awoke after the operation. "The scarring is pervasive. I was unable to remove any of it. Likely your heart has been sick for a long time." He had no idea how long. "The good news is that we successfully repaired your leaking valves."

I would no longer be confined to bed and a wheelchair. In fact, I could start attending cardiac rehab—an exercise class designed for heart patients. It was located at our local hospital and attended by a cardiac nurse and a physical therapist, who would monitor my heart-rate while I exercised.

While all my heart experiences were happening, Bob's ex-wife, Mariana, and her fiancé, Michael, were having a somewhat parallel experience. Michael had also succumbed to heart failure, of a different kind, and also needed cardiac rehab.

Concepts I'd had about the line between old relationships and new ones were healing. My physical heart was still getting larger—dangerously so—but my spiritual heart was growing, too.

So I accepted Michael's offer to pick me up three times a week and go to rehab together. It was a leap of faith, because at first I wasn't sure how we would get along. It turned out I had nothing to worry about. Michael was as easy-going as could be, a good conversationalist, and an all-around nice guy. He had become an angel of sorts, who helped me get to rehab class until I was able to drive there on my own.

9

ANGELS AND HARD EVIDENCE

I've been gifted with many angels on my transplant journey. My first "real" angel was the woman who appeared next to me outside the clinic where I'd gone for blood work. This was months before the open-heart surgery when any movement made me feel ill.

The building didn't have wheelchair access, so I had crept step-by-labored-step to get inside. When we were done, I had to repeat the process to get back out. I thought I'd never make it to the parking lot. It wasn't just utter weakness; it was the terribly sick feeling you get when your cells simply do not have enough oxygen to function. As a result, your body feels like a cement block, and you can hardly breathe.

I was standing outside while Bob was getting the car.

The woman appeared from nowhere and put her arm around me to help me stay upright.

"God is with you. God is with you."

She repeated the phrase over and over again. Her words kept my knees from buckling and my blood pressure from dropping out. Her loving presence was a priceless gift that gave me more than strength and comfort. It was proof that I was being taken care of every step of the way.

After the open heart surgery in January, 2004, I enjoyed several good months. I was able to visit with my two youngest daughters at the same time, I was able to drive, I resumed writing, we vacationed in Maine that summer, and life appeared to be getting back to normal.

That autumn, my health started to wane. I was tired sooner at night, and nausea kept me from eating well. I experienced more light-headedness, chest tightness, and palpitations. I no longer had the stamina to drive, and although I was still doing cardiac rehab three times a week, I hadn't been able to improve any of my numbers for over two months. More importantly, I felt something big was impending. Dear friends invited us to a party and, although I really wanted to go, my inner guidance invoked a survival instinct that told me to stay home. So I did.

At my next doctor's appointment in October, 2004, I mentioned my symptoms.

"I understand you aren't feeling well," my doctor said. "According to the readout from your I.C.D. [internal cardiac defibrillator], there's no evidence that anything has worsened. So there's nothing I can do."

My doctors needed hard evidence?

Soon enough, they were going to get it.

A few weeks later, I was writing at my desk when I had an odd feeling that my blood pressure was going to drop. Usually when I got this feeling, I would have time to reach my bed so I could lie down. This time, I sensed the drop was coming too fast for that.

"Call 911." This inner directive—clearly the voice of my spiritual guide—came loud and clear.

The next thing I knew, the phone was ringing. I opened my eyes. I was lying on the floor with the phone beside me. It took a few rings before I realized I needed to answer it.

"This is the 911 operator. We just received a call from your phone number. Is everything okay?"

This resulted in yet another ride to the emergency room, so I knew the routine. This was the first time I had passed out—another clue something was going wrong.

On November 29, 2004, I got the same dreadful feeling once again.

Before I tell you what happened, I'd like to mention an objection some people have given me about working with gemstones. They tell me that in a crisis, they feel they should call on their spiritual guide first—not reach for a gemstone. I agree. And I'm not sure why they would think otherwise. In this case, I did neither.

I called Bob.

"I'll be there as fast as possible," he said. "I'll take you to the emergency room."

Then I thought about my spiritual guide and sang HU for a few minutes.

The lightheadedness passed so I gathered a few things that I wanted to bring to the hospital—lotion, tissues, and pajamas.

Suddenly, the feeling returned.

I felt myself losing consciousness. What did I have to do to survive? My thoughts raced.

I lay on the bed—it was better than falling on the floor.

A second later: BHAM!

My I.C.D. went off for the first time. My body convulsed.

They say it feels like a kick from a horse. They don't say it's a kick from the front, the back, and the side all at the same time. Another way to describe it is like a bolt of lightning going off in your chest.

BHAM!

It went off a second time.

Then a third time.

I called my neighbor, Jack, who was at my side in seconds. He called 911 for me.

BHAM.

His wife, Lorraine, arrived to lend her support, too.

The experience was like being on a roller coaster and it was maddening. I felt myself drifting into the Peaceful Place and then BHAM, I'd get kicked awake, my body would jerk and then all was quiet once again. I was back in the bedroom with my friends as though nothing had happened—except for the telltale pain leftover in my chest.

It took the paramedics over twenty minutes to arrive. While we waited, the I.C.D. continued to jolt me every few minutes, so finding solace in the gray zone wasn't an option. The unit would go off twenty-one times by the time I finally got to the hospital. I would be told that this set a record (which I would soon break, and which many others after me would break yet again).

As the paramedics wheeled me into the ambulance I was given a knowing—clear as a bell—that I would not be returning home without a new heart.

In the ambulance, the I.C.D. kicks grew stronger. The paramedics explained that the unit was detecting that its previous voltage was not enough, so it automatically shifted to a stronger dosage of electricity. I could barely handle it. In desperation, I called out to my spiritual guide—inwardly, of course, so I would not have to explain my plea to the paramedics.

"What is this about?" I wanted to know.

I received an unexpected reply. The image of Harold appeared in living color before me. Since I was lying down and looking up, his image appeared on the ceiling of the ambulance.

He said, "The doctors need irrefutable evidence that you need a new heart. Bear with it."

It had been a long time since I'd had such a clear and vivid spiritual experience. Rather than revel in the blessing, my circumstances required that I take it in stride. I had asked a question, and my spiritual guide had answered. I would trust what he said and bear the pain.

When we arrived at the emergency room, a doctor was standing outside to meet us. I could tell by the expression on his face that he hadn't a clue what to do, and this was confirmed when he did nothing (except call another doctor for advice). Granted, I'm sure they did not get cases like mine on a regular basis. At least not in 2004 when I.C.D.s were relatively new devices.

Furthermore, they could not get a line into the veins in my arm. I told them to cut off my jeans and use one in my groin. They said they could not do that until they were sure they were unable get a vein in my arm. I knew it was a waste of time, yet I had to let them go through their protocol. Soon enough, my jeans were cut with my permission, and an I.V. inserted into a vein in my groin.

Meanwhile, I was slipping in and out of consciousness. I was aware that the room was crowded with attendants, who were working on me. To my left, a woman was gently stroking my hand, telling me I was okay.

How did she know to say that? Usually people say, "You're going to be okay," which means, right now, you're not okay. I hated to hear that because I wanted to agree with the mindset that I was okay, and then my body would follow that truth.

Looking back and judging from where her voice was coming from, she must have been no more than three feet tall, and somehow nestled among all the others who were working on me.

She was the second angel that I was aware of since the heart failure.

When I became stable, my I.C.D. stopped firing, and everyone left me alone. I'm going to mention what happened next in hope that someone will change policies so it never happens to anyone else. I was left naked, with nothing covering my body. This in itself didn't bother me, and I didn't care that I was alone. After all, I had enough monitors hooked up to me that if anything stopped working, the staff would know immediately. I do not remember being cold or warm, as I was mostly out of consciousness, and so it didn't matter.

After what seemed a long time, a man with a kind voice came to sit by my right side, near my head, and he asked me how I was doing. I tried to answer him but could not move my mouth. This was because I was out of my body, perched somewhere above my head, watching over myself.

Then the attending doctor came in—the one I'd previously pegged as oblivious. I watched him look at me. He asked the man to my right if I was unconscious and didn't get a definitive reply. So the doctor pinched my nipple.

In my own defense, I rushed back into my body and managed to groan.

"Why did you do that?" the kind man asked.

The doctor said it was a foolproof way to find out if I was awake or not.

The kind man then ordered someone to cover me. I wished he'd punched the doctor, too. Right smack in the nose.

Had I been awake I would have placed the punch elsewhere... well, actually... in that case I would not have been in this situation.

There must be a more dignified, respectful way to find out if a woman is unconscious.

10

ALIVE AFTER DEATH

I was admitted to the hospital's intensive care unit and given intravenous lidocaine to keep my heart from going into v-tach. The lidocaine worked.

Dad flew in as soon as he'd heard I was back in the hospital. He and Bob kept me company all day long, chatting and telling funny stories. I told my one and only joke about my friend's embarrassing reaction to my "implant."

I was growing stronger, and on the fifth day, the doctors decided to cut back the lidocaine to eventually wean me of it and send me home. I was sitting in a chair beside my bed in the intensive care unit, involved in a conversation with Dad and Bob. Mid-sentence, the familiar caffeine-buzz sensation returned.

I looked at my father. "Here we go again," I said.

My room was suddenly crowded with nurses, who helped me back into bed. My I.C.D. fired, and I felt myself losing consciousness. The medical staff busily tried to keep me alive as the I.C.D. fired four more times.

Afterward, Bob told me that he and Dad watched my vital-signs on the monitor by the nurses' station. Soon, they flat-lined.

"What's going on?" Bob asked someone who left my room.

"We lost her."

Yet the nurses who surrounded me did not give up.

*   *   *

The transition to the other side of life was as easy as blinking. My eyes closed in one world and opened in another. In one moment I was suffering from the pain of the horse-like kicks and a horrible feeling of sickness. In the next, complete Peace.

This time the light I'd once seen on the horizon in the gray zone engulfed me. I did not leave my hospital room to go to it. It came to me. No longer was I lying down, I was sitting upright in the bed. Instead of being surrounded by nurses, my company included several spiritual masters I had come to know and love.

Gopal Das, a master from ancient Egypt, with long white hair bleached by the Light of God, stood at my feet. A Persian master in a maroon robe, Shamus-i-Tabriz, sat by my right side. At my right shoulder stood Rebazar. At my left, was my friend Fubbi Quantz, who had visited me as a child, and next to him, Kentucky-born Peddar Zaskq, wearing khaki pants and a blue shirt. To my left and a short distance away watched Yaubl Sacabi, a bare-headed master, also in maroon.

Each had a personal message for me of spiritual significance. I can share what Shamus told me. He said that everything I had experienced inwardly in the past was true. This was a revelation of sorts because I had doubted certain past-life recalls, and especially those experiences with the gemstone guardians.

The American master, Harold Klemp, stood behind a curtain of shimmering blue light just a few feet away from the foot of my bed. The curtain consisted of millions of tiny bright blue stars. Instinctively, I knew what it was. It was the portal to heaven. Was I ready to pass? It seemed as though I had a choice. What would it be like if I moved through it? My curiosity propelled me forward.

The next thing knew, I was witnessing my memorial service. I was a pair of eyes hovering near the blue stained-glass star in the ceiling above the audience in our temple's sanctuary. I saw how my death affected my friends, and I could hear their thoughts and feelings about my life and my passing. I was respected and loved, but my memory would eventually fade. That's how it goes, and I was okay with that.

I also saw how my death affected Bob, my parents, and my five children both now and as they grew to adulthood. For them my memory was not so easily healed, and my permanent absence gave new shape to their pain.

Outside of my body, I felt no emotion or sentimentality— only compassion and love. I tried to make words with this compassion and whisper them into my loved ones' ears. I urged them to move on with life and to grow with my memory as something that ignited them to succeed, rather than something that weighed upon them. I urged them to find happiness.

When I could do no more for them—and they could receive no more from me—my attention lifted back to heaven. I stood on a well-manicured lawn beside a golden temple. I was about fourth in line before a great white angel who seemed three times my height. When it was my turn, the angel read from the book that he held, and gave me my assignment:

"You will explore the higher levels of heaven, locate temples there and then bring back certain information. You shall transcribe what you learn."

I had a purpose here? I cannot tell you how reassuring that was.

This was, literally, my dream job. It gave me permission to travel freely among the heavenly planes. I could explore answers that could be found only there, and then make them available to others. This job allowed me to research and discover. It served me and let me serve others. It let me express my passion for living, challenged my creativity, and demanded my very best. Joy abounded. What more could I want?

I recorded what I learned while seated in a vast library with an immensely tall ceiling. Every inch of the room represented someone's divinely inspired creativity, from the mosaic wood floor to the finely carved furniture to the intricately painted ceiling. Stacks of books reached twenty feet high, and I was also aware of technology that I could not identify.

My first journal entry while sitting in this library recounted my journey from the hospital to heaven. I wrote:

I am drawn upward, as though on a swiftly rising elevator. The ceiling—a limitation I can sense but not see—recedes as I move up. It seems to open, broaden, and expand as I do.

Where am I? I know that I am exactly where I need to be. Clearly, I am centered within eternity, fully present in its middle where I am stationed as the observer. I am also everywhere. I exist in every square inch of creation.

I feel an undeniable Presence. I am among countless others like myself, and also I am the only being in existence, alone with the One.

I realize these descriptions seem contradictory. During my experience they made perfect, beautiful sense. I continued to write:

The one unmistakable constant is the Light and Sound. There is no darkness here and music is everywhere. The Light sings. Or perhaps the all-pervasive Sound produces this brightness. This world is extremely, palpably, deeply silent, except for the Sound, which fills my ears and every atom of my being—whatever I am. I have no sense of having a body or any form at all.

I became aware that I was writing on something that looked like paper. Somehow, it transferred my words directly into a large tome that rested on the table beside me. I held an ink pen, and miraculously (if you've seen my illegible handwriting), the resulting cursive was elegant and perfect.

The Sound's rhythm enters my awareness subtly at first. Then it grows until I become aware that I am riding the undulating waves of a vast ocean. I feel as though I am a tiny tree that has been uprooted and tossed into the sea. The water's molecules rip away any soil that my roots still cling to—all my attachments and everything that I hold dear or that remind me of life on Earth. The purge is exhilarating. With every bit of soil that washes away, I feel freer. More Me.

Meanwhile the leaves of my uprooted tree have nothing to shield them from the Light. I am scorched by the fire, yet also sated by the cool water beneath me. These sensations do not produce pain, but delight, and an ever-increasing sense of freedom that does not stop growing.

Eventually, the difference between one degree of freedom and the next dissolves. There is nothing left to wash away. I am free.

The memories ended and my attention wandered to the table at which I sat. It was made of a single slab of wood. I was entranced by its beauty. Its edge must have been as wide as my hand and along it someone had carved a series of scenes that told the story of the wood's history.

I got up to walk around the table and examine the intricate engravings. The first depicted a person planting the seed of the tree, whose wood would eventually become the table. Following scenes told of the changes in the landscape surrounding the tree that occurred with each passing decade, the buildings that grew up around the tree, the animals who lived on the tree or in it, and the people who visited it and were inspired by it. The tree's story continued with its death and the many ways its wood was used. Next an account of those who sat at this table, inspired by it. I saw myself depicted there and felt flushed with the improbability of this record and turned my attention immediately away. Even in heaven there were things that stretched my mind more than I could bear.

I looked up at the ceiling and saw more improbable beauty. It was artistry that must have inspired Michelangelo. These heavenly scenes were populated by angels enacting kind deeds and miracles. Although the colorful murals were a hundred feet away, whenever I focused on them, they would appear close, as though my eyesight was somehow telescopic.

After marveling at this otherworldly talent, it was time to return to my work. I sat back down, picked up the pen, and returned to new memories.

My attention is captured by the waves of sound. Although I can just as easily describe them as rippling ribbons of light. Whatever they are, their intelligence is unmistakable.

As though inviting me to get to know them, the ribbons fill my attention. The ocean is now a multitude of uncountable ribbon-like waves. I play by riding one of them, like on a surfboard, and then I try riding many at once.

I am sublimely content to be in this world of Light and Sound. I know I am absorbing the experience of being here and also being absorbed by it. I know that it is changing me.

Can I ride the waves of Light forever? Possibly, except that this sea of divine intelligence has a propensity for curiosity, and I had become curious. I wanted to investigate this wondrous Light and Sound that surrounded and permeated me, that both held me and set me free—that granted both stillness and unstoppable activity—that gave me life.

Curiosity opened the door, and something shifted. My awareness moved away from being interconnected with my surroundings, and I became separate and apart from that which

encompassed and pervaded me. Self-aware, I knew I was dis-
tinctly and uniquely alive and capable of choice. My choice
defined the Light and it became knowledge.

In this state I could simply understand anything that I
gave my attention to.

Then, as though waking up from a dream, the scene shifted
again. The light took form. I was now standing on a well-manicured lawn, outside a golden temple, waiting in line before a
great angel, who was handing out assignments.

* * *

Time passed in my heavenly lifetime. I continued to research
the higher planes and write what I learned into my journal in
the great library. It seemed as though I was there for months, if
not years. One day, I was sitting at my table, carefully transcribing some age-old truths I'd uncovered in some corner of light in
some higher world. A tap on my shoulder roused me.

"It's time to reincarnate."

I stopped, confused, and turned to face the Great Angel who
had come for me.

"I do not need to reincarnate anymore. I have earned the
right to be in this world and never to return to Earth."

"You have more to learn about love."

"I do?"

I knew my reply and the innocence behind it confirmed he
was correct.

"There is always more to learn about love."

"I can learn it here." I glanced at the forest of bookcases that
formed a comfortable cocoon around me.

"What about your spiritual goals?"

My deepest desire was spiritual mastership and my goal was
God-Realization.

Having heard my thoughts, the Great Angel asked, "What do these mean to you?"

I thought a moment. "It means having such a close connection with Spirit that every atom of my being sings with God's love. It means my life is guided every step by the Divine, and that it inspires and ignites divine love in everyone I meet."

"You know these goals are best realized in the Physical World, where the mirror of karma reflects most accurately and immediately. The physical incarnation is a gift. Treasure it, and take care of it."

I knew what he said was true. I had a long way to go to reach my spiritual goals. I had more to learn about love.

I had to go back.

But reincarnation is such a hassle.

Spiritual masters I recognized and loved, and a few I did not know, now joined the Great Angel to discuss my situation. Looking back, it reminded me of a team huddle during a game of American football.

As a result of the meeting, the master Fubbi Quantz led me to a waist-high basket, leaned over it, and ruffled through it. It seemed as though he was searching through a pile of clothing, and nothing looked as though it was going to fit. He was looking for the right karma for me to bear in my next life. The karma would anchor me in the Physical World and keep me there until I learned all that I could.

"There is an alternative," said Rebazar. I picked up his telepathic communication to Fubbi Quantz: The previous body I had occupied could still be revived. It required only a slight adjustment of my place on the time track. It would be an easy thing for them to do.

"It won't be easy to live out her life in her old body," Fubbi said.

"She has worked through so much of her karma already," Rebazar said. "It would be a shame to give her yet another burden just so she can reincarnate."

Rebazar was rooting for me!

The two masters discussed things privately for a moment and then seemed to come to a conclusion.

*　*　*

The surgical spotlights overhead blinded my eyes, and the cardiopulmonary resuscitation that someone was performing on my chest immediately stopped. I groaned from the pain of the external defibrillator. I wondered how many times they had shocked my body this time.

Once I was stable, all the nurses filed out of my room to attend to someone else who now needed their care more than I did.

Dad and Bob came in.

"Don't touch me," I said with as much force as I could muster. I knew Bob would have wanted to hug me. I was so fragile, and my gift of life was not yet set in stone. I knew that one touch would have stimulated my heart into another v-tach storm that I knew I could not recover from. Thankfully, he obeyed.

I could tell both Dad and Bob were very glad to have me back. I tried to explain to Bob what had happened. "I came back because there's more I need to learn about love," I whispered.

Bob leaned over me to get as close as he could without touching me. "You're the most loving being I know."

How could he understand? I didn't have the strength to explain it.

*　*　*

"Would you like more morphine?" a nurse asked.

More? My mind started turning. "Did you give me some already?"

"Yes, for the pain."

I was not feeling any pain at the moment and was about to say so when a feeling of dread rose within me. At the time, I believed that morphine was a hallucinogen (although when researching this book I learned this is not necessarily so). What if that fantastic experience I'd just had—which seemed more real than real—was simply the illusions incurred by morphine?

"Yes, please."

Yes, give me more so that I can return to that lovely place. Give me another dose so that I can prove to my spiteful, cynical, doubting mind that the blessings I'd just witnessed were products of my imagination, liberated by a mere drug. Let the majesty and miracle of my experience return so that I can see it for the illusion it truly was.

I watched the second hand of the clock on the wall turn countless cycles until midnight.

In 1992, my best girlfriend, Natalie, had foreseen her death from cancer at midnight of a certain day. At that precise moment, she departed. The clock fell off the wall and broke, immortalizing the hour. I expected the same would happen to me.

Midnight came and went.

Okay then, two o'clock would be my death, I decided. The masters would again come around my bed and invite me through the curtain of blue light. I yearned to be back within the worlds of light, surrounded by peace and knowing. I imagined being there as desperately as I could.

Two o'clock passed, as did three o'clock and four. The masters never arrived. I couldn't even pretend they were there.

Yet that morning I awoke to beautiful music. It was a balm, like honey nectar, a healing salve. For the smallest moment I thought I might have been back in the Peaceful Place. The pain, sickness, and weak feeling told me I was not.

What about that beautiful sound?

As my awareness emerged from sleep, I realized the woman who had come into my room to mop the floor was humming. I clung to her music as though it was breath itself. She was about to leave.

"Please don't leave."

She said something to me in Spanish.

"Your humming is healing."

She smiled and mopped the floor again, humming louder this time.

She was an angel who returned every day to mop my floor and sing to me. I thanked her each time.

A few days later they moved me to the other side of the intensive care unit, to a room that had windows. They wanted me to acclimate to the sun, so that my sleep cycle could normalize. The room had fewer ceiling tiles. I know, because I spent a lot of time counting them.

11

I LEARN ABOUT SPECTRUMS

*I*n mid-November 2004, while I was still in the I.C.U. and a few days after my near-death experience, the doctors wanted to try to fix my irregular heartbeat, which was an underlying cause of my heart failure. They suggested a procedure called "ablation." Ablation has helped many people who suffer from arrhythmia.

The procedure took place in a cold operating room. Even colder were the strips of electrical tape they stuck to my front, back, and sides.

"To keep me from falling apart?" I joked.

"Just in case we have to use the defibrillator," a nurse said.

Ugh, that good-old defibrillator.

Time passes instantly when you're under general anesthesia and I awoke in agony. Obviously, they had used the defibrillator. I learned they had shocked me more than once. The horse had kicked my back, side, and front repeatedly. Even still, waves of pain rippled down my legs. Every part of me deeply ached.

As they rolled me out of the operating room, my one comfort was an invisible little yellow bird that sat on my shoulder. My eyes were closed and still I could see him—as though I had a pair of eyes a few feet above my body. I could feel his warm feathers against my cheek and hear his cheerful chirping. Nothing could have comforted me more.

Before the procedure I'd asked my spiritual guide to be with me and somehow to show me that he was there. This bird was my answer.

Was the bird illusion? In that moment I didn't care. Sometimes you have to accept the gifts just as they are—just as you perceive them—and not let your mind take your comfort away.

"We kept losing her blood pressure," I overheard the doctor say to Bob. "We had to revive her several times. The procedure was not successful."

All the pain for nothing.

In the recovery room, I felt sick and emptied my stomach. The bile smelled sour and disgusting. The contents poured warm over my shoulder and down my back. Bob and the nurse cleaned me up while I tried to hide from the pain in the solitude of sleep.

The yellow bird chirped on.

A few days later the doctor wanted to try the same procedure once again.

"It didn't work the first time," I told Bob.

He was sitting beside my hospital bed, and looked up from his magazine. "If the doctor gets it right, you can be cured."

Did I want to go through the torment of another failed ablation? No. But it was my next step and I had to take it.

So, we repeated the performance—and the finale. When I awoke in the cold operating room, another bird, a blue one, sang to me on my left shoulder. The yellow one chirped on my right. Each nestled their heads against my cheeks, and I reveled in the sweet comfort of their soft feathers.

"How are you?" the doctor asked as they wheeled me into the recovery room.

"Pain," I groaned. "Everywhere."

"I'm sorry I hurt you."

I'll never forget the sincerity of his words. The procedure had again failed, and yet he had given his best. More, he had given his apology. It was heartfelt and touched me deeply. It made the aftermath easier to bear. I'm sure his malpractice insurance company would have frowned on the gesture. I applaud him for it.

Recovering from this second procedure took much longer. The first night in the intensive care unit I was a mess. Pain wracked my body, and I felt anxious and unsettled. Then—in precious moments—I would dip into sleep, shed my shell of misery, and enter a world of dazzling light and color.

The first time this happened, I was surrounded by countless translucent spheres nearly as large as I was. The spheres reminded me of soap bubbles and each displayed a spectrum of color.

The spheres represented entire lifetimes—my lifetimes. I looked into one and saw it was packed with more bubbles. These were the experiences contained within the lifetime. If I looked into any of these tiny bubbles I could see even smaller ones. These represented the components that made up the experience: the thoughts, words, actions, and emotions. These had spectrums too.

I felt elated when I realized that everything had a spectrum!

Spectrums within spectrums comprised all of life!

Spectrums were the secret of creation. They explained how Light and Sound worked together to manifest all things. Only a Soul in its pure form could approach and receive pure spiritual light. In contrast, the body required that light to be broken down into its components. These were the seven colors of the rainbow: red, orange, yellow, green, blue, indigo, and purple.

A nurse entered my room to check on me, and my awareness hurtled back into my body. My stomach emptied and proceeded to do so every ten minutes for the next few hours. I felt incredibly restless and could hear myself babbling nonsense.

When I was relatively stable, the nurse left, and I drifted into another moment of peace. Again I was outside the body. It was as though the dip back into physical hell had never happened. I refocused on the spectrums and saw them from a different viewpoint.

This time I focused on the smallest most essential spectrums—those of atoms. Stepping back, I could see they organized themselves into larger spectrums—those of molecules. These were encompassed by the spectrums of cells, which were enveloped by those of the organs. A larger spectrum, which signified the body, incorporated all the others. The emotion-body spectrum encompassed all of this. Beyond that, the memory and mind bodies occupied progressively larger bubbles with ever more encompassing spectrums. The largest spectrum contained the sum of all. This spectrum encompassed a person's whole being.

The spectrums drew me into themselves, as though inviting me into their hidden truths. I felt as though more secrets of the mechanics of the universe were going to be revealed. I looked more closely and carefully at the spectrums and I found something I did not expect to see.

The surprise forced my attention back to my body, which began sweating profusely. My sheets were soaked. I was nauseous again, and my head hurt so much I could hardly stand it.

"No pain meds until you stop vomiting," my nurse said. She and an assistant changed my linens and gave me a fresh hospital gown.

"I could use a sip of water." My mouth felt like sandpaper.

"Keep your stomach calm a little while first."

I pleaded and she gave me a chip of ice. What sweet relief.

I fell back into the colors.

My discovery: Spectrums consisted of two parts!

I heard someone say, "This secret of the spectrums forms the basis of several universal laws. The law of attraction is one, the law of opposites another, and the law of karma yet another."

"Who said that?"

It was a female voice.

I looked around for its source and found her. She had long brown hair, orange-toned skin, and her body was draped in layers of sheer orange fabric that glistened. Where had I seen her before?

She stood at the front of an open-air room lined with school desks. The single wall behind her held a small waterfall and flowering vines. The floor beneath us was a marble platform situated in a large garden surrounded by nature. The room's ceiling was supported by white columns. Beyond them I could see a lake with mountains in the distance. I felt as though I had awoken in a Maxfield Parrish painting.

I was the lone student in the class. "Each half of the spectrum contains all seven colors," the woman said. She held up her left hand. "One half is the spectrum that resides in all things. It represents root cause. We call it the resident spectrum." She held up her right hand. "The other half of the spectrum represents effect. We call it the experience spectrum."

She moved her right hand toward her left. "The resident spectrum draws the effect spectrum into a person's life. Cause attracts effect."

"Are you talking about karma?"

"Yes." Her hands were clasped.

This was remarkable! It meant that karma could be explained in terms of spectrums.

"As the colors in a resident spectrum attract an experience spectrum, karma is worked out. When the experience spectrum perfectly completes the resident spectrum, then karma is resolved.

The spectrums should then move out of a person's life, to be stored in her karmic records."

She sat down in a seat next to mine, and continued, "Resident spectrums are inherent in all things. They're the ones we start with. In the East, they might be called the "adi karma." The resident spectrums of cells draw nutrients, water, and oxygen, along with the spectrums that accompany them. The resident spectrum of the entire body draws the spectrums of emotions, thoughts, and actions.

"How strongly and swiftly a resident spectrum draws an experience spectrum depends upon a single color in the resident spectrum. This color is present in least amount. Therefore, it has the most to gain by attracting an experience spectrum—for then that color will not be deficient any more. Hence, of all the seven colors in the spectrum, this one has the greatest magnetic pull."

My attention was drawn partially back to the intensive care unit. What ensued was a profound split in my awareness. On the one hand, I was struggling with my body's needs and discomforts, and on the other, I was contemplating the spectrums.

I wondered about the spectrum that was directing the experiences I was having now. Which color was present in least amount? It was indeed calling experiences to me—but way too strongly for my liking.

"The color most responsible for attracting life experiences is called the main color ray," the woman in orange told me. "It is the color present in least amount in your whole-being spectrum. In your case, you have so many spectrums on so many levels that have become deficient in color, that they are powerfully calling experience spectrums toward you in multiples."

"How did they become so deficient?"

"Neglect."

"Neglect?"

"You have been avoiding your destiny."

I didn't want to hear that.

Another round of sweating must have elevated my heart rate and alerted the nurse, who returned to change my linens once again. When she was finished, I didn't want to be left alone.

"Can you sit with me?" I begged.

"For a little while." She brought some paperwork into my room to work on.

"I can't sleep."

"You'll be fine. Just rest."

Right. I will be fine. Right now I wasn't fine. I babbled about who knows what.

"Am I your worst patient?"

She thought a moment and then smiled, "Top five." It was a lighthearted moment.

Never before had I witnessed such compassion. This nurse taught me what it means to give fully and selflessly. I could also feel myself being humbled by the pain. It was softening my rigid attitudes and beliefs, making me more capable of accepting truth. This prepared me to learn more.

I dipped back into the altered state and watched the spectrum bubbles interact with each other as though immersed in play. I watched how my main color ray navigated the bubble of my whole being among all the other whole-being bubbles that existed in my life—and right now, these were the nurses who took care of me. I also saw how the main color ray drove the smaller bubbles of experiences into my life, which were associated with the pain, discomfort, and anxiety.

Curiously, the main ray could do more than attract experiences, it could also organize them and ensure they came in an orderly manner. If the main ray was not so depleted, it could make sure that my whole-being bubble was positioned perfectly among all others both small and large. In this way, karma could be resolved efficiently. I would get only the experiences I needed to complete the resident spectrums that I was responsible for— the ones I had created through my own actions or inactions.

I returned to the inner-world classroom, curious to learn more. I also wanted to know how to replenish my main ray.

"Without a main ray, a Soul would attract experiences willy-nilly, without reason or purpose," the woman in orange said. "Your main ray is ensuring that you have the experiences you require. It will also attract the resources you need to meet those experiences and see them through.

"Spectrums comprise all of life," she emphasized. "AND they drive all life experiences!"

I thought about my spectrum bubbles and recalled how much their colors varied. One spectrum had a little more yellow than another, another had a little more red or blue. The uneven amounts reminded me of the jagged edge of a key.

She said, "If you change the amount of the colors in your key even slightly, then a different door will open for you."

"How can I change the spectrum my body is experiencing now, to feel less sick?"

"Work with your main color ray."

I could hear the command in her voice.

Wasn't my main color ray indigo? The memory pushed itself forward. I had learned this years before when I was working with gemstones. I would wear the gemstone called "Indigo" which is a rare type of Sodalite that is translucent and gemlike. It would nourish my body and aura with the indigo color ray.

If somehow I could give myself more indigo ray right now, then the experience spectrums would not be thundering into my life as they were doing now in the intensive care unit. The

uncomfortable reactions I was having to the latest ablation procedure would ease.

I imagined an ocean of indigo light.

And then I jumped in.

12

WHY I STOPPED WORKING
WITH GEMSTONES

$\mathcal{I}$ntensive care units, in my experience, are not a place to bring gemstones, nor anything of value. Yet, if you've been wearing them, your body is familiar with their healing energies and it is possible to invite those healing energies to you, wherever you may be. Then, even though your necklaces are not physically present with you, they can serve you.

This ability to transcend space fascinates me. In the world of energy medicine, it's very real. I can be talking to a customer on the phone and, with her permission, bring gemstones into her energy field, and if she is sensitive enough, as most people are, she will feel the difference between one necklace and another. We do not need to be in the same room. Not even on the same continent.

Had I been actively walking my gemstone journey at this time, which ones would I have chosen, and how?

First, I would have identified what exactly I wanted help with. The more clearly you state your intention, the better. In the I.C.U., I might have chosen the profound weakness, the overall feeling of sickness, or my inability to sleep on a regular cycle.

Then I would have tuned into my collection of gemstones or thought about them with a grateful and open heart and asked

97

which ones would support me in this moment. In some way the ones that could help would have made themselves known. The image of one or two necklaces might have come to mind, or just their names might have popped into my head. Maybe, they would have remained nameless, and I would just have felt their presence.

I might have formally invited these necklaces in—even if I was unable to identify them. I'd imagine their energies seeping into my body and radiating into my aura. At the very least, I would have been comforted to know that my physical progress was being supported energetically. I certainly would have felt the sense of empowerment that comes when you are able to have some control over your own situation—something that rarely happens in a hospital.

It's best to call upon those gemstones that you have had personal experience with. Either you've worn them, or your Gemstone Therapy practitioner has used them on you during a session. This way, your body knows exactly what energetic frequencies you are calling in. Otherwise, if you call upon a gemstone that you have not personally experienced—say therapeutic-quality Morganite for emotional support—you'll only be able to draw upon the mental concept that you have of this gemstone. This concept may comprise only a fraction of the gem's true capabilities. Of course, this may be enough in some cases.

During my stay in the hospital, I often got phone calls from my parents, brothers, and children. When I got a call from my son Aaron, who was then age fifteen, we got past the small talk quickly. He had questions on his mind.

"Why did you change your name when you and my dad got divorced?"

Indeed I had chosen both a new first and last name. I said, 'Sometimes when two people get together, things don't work out as they expect them to. My life married to your father had become like a shoe too small. I felt I had grown away from needing the experiences the marriage provided and changing my name was a way to find my own identity.'"

I felt too embarrassed to tell him that my need to re-establish this identity was due to the overuse of channeling. Even after we had published our book about the gemstone guardians, I was still channeling the inner-world doctor.

Without telling my son this part of the story, I could not seem to get across to him how important it was for me to reestablish and discover myself—apart from any being I had once channeled. Part of the problem was that I didn't really know who I was. I had gotten married and pregnant before I graduated college. I'd had no time living on my own to become comfortable with myself, sure of who I was, and clear about what I liked and didn't like and what I would and would not allow. Channeling other beings compounded this problem. Worse, their spectrums got mixed up with my own. I lost sight of my identity and it was excruciating.

He then asked, "Why did you stop working with gemstones?"

This was a bigger question. There were many reasons. The most obvious was that because I could no longer be married to his father, I could no longer do business with him either. Furthermore, upon our divorce in 1992, I had signed a non-compete agreement. After this agreement expired, I still had no interest in working with gemstones, so I never did. These were the reasons I gave him. There were more.

Back in 1988, testimonials from people who loved working with the gemstones poured in. So did the backlash. People whom I respected had some discomforting things to say about my work and about me. I believe David shielded me from much of it. Nonetheless, I got the message loud and clear.

In 1991, we were attending a seminar when I crossed paths with a certain woman in the convention center lobby. I respected her very much, and my heart opened when I saw her. I was about to smile in recognition when the encounter took an unexpected turn.

The woman gave me a penetrating stare, backed with boatloads of judgment.

I knew she had heard about our work and now clearly communicated her disapproval. Her expression ingrained itself in my mind's eye and haunted me for years. It made me doubt everything I was doing. In a word, I felt shattered.

Obviously, she and others felt that working with gemstones was nothing short of sacrilegious and that channeling was wrong.

It turned out they were right—in part. It was the channeling that would prove dangerous and destructive for me, not the gemstone work. Had I stopped channeling after the guardian interviews, I believe everything would have been fine. Gemstone Therapy would have spread much sooner into the alternative healing community and by now be better recognized as a legitimate complementary modality.

Instead, every night, I continued to channel Hahn.

After I put the children to sleep, David and I would sit on the couch in our bedroom and meet with Hahn. David asked his council about every aspect of the business, from pricing to marketing to hiring new employees. The two became friends, and they enjoyed their conversations together. Hahn's advice always seemed wise and sensible.

Increasingly, I felt left out of the equation. I felt as though my input, thoughts, and ideas were never asked for and were belittled if I offered them. As you can imagine, this was the recipe for marriage disaster. As the months went by, I began to resent all the time that David spent with Hahn.

When I complained, David insisted the conversations were essential for the company's survival.

I couldn't argue that.

Had I been self-worthy enough, loved and respected myself enough to lay clear guidelines for the channeling, circumstances might have turned out differently, although I doubt it. Looking back, it was clear that my mission with the gemstones could only be fulfilled if I were fully in charge of its manifestation. I would need to captain my own ship.

And so the marriage unraveled.

The channeling dimmed the spiritual light within me. Each time I came out of the trance, I felt more out of touch with myself. It was as though I was a boat lost on a stormy sea, without any instruments to tell me which way was north. My food wasn't digesting properly, I couldn't think straight, I felt disconnected from my children, and I lost contact with the inner masters. No longer did I see Rebazar out of the corner of my eye, there to protect and guide me.

I was so off course, so disconnected, that I justified walking out on three young children.

I truly believed that to survive, I had no other choice.

I was really, really out of balance.

By stepping away from the gemstone world and changing my name, I thought I could shed the stigma, find my own identity, and move forward spiritually. This was paramount. My spirituality felt like a life-preserver; there was nothing I wanted more.

Abruptly and necessarily, my work with David ended. The book we had written together went out of print. I gladly gave David my copyrights to the gemstone work we had done together. I have never regretted this decision because our gemstone business, which he continued, supported our three children.

To be clear, I place no blame for my leaving on anyone except myself. I respected David, and I still do, and he had respected me and my abilities. He had originally listed me as principal partner in the banking and legal organization of our company. It was I who was unable to fill the shoes given to me. Nor did I want them by the time of our divorce.

When I left the marriage, I truly believed my involvement with gemstones had ended forever.

At some point before I left, I remember dreaming I had boarded a powerful steam locomotive. As the train pulled away from the station I looked back and saw I had left something precious on the platform. I wanted dearly to get off and get it—but was too afraid to jump.

13

AN ASSIGNMENT I DO NOT WANT

A few days later, they moved me out of the intensive care unit. I had a room to myself in the cardiac wing where I would continue my recovery.

The room was sparsely decorated with an end-table, food tray, medical equipment, and a television set, which I didn't even have the strength to watch. In the evenings I would gaze out the window that overlooked a bridge. Dreamily, I watched the headlights of cars zooming over it. I envied the drivers, who seemed in such a hurry to get somewhere. In contrast, I was going nowhere—so it seemed.

My daughter, AriaRay, had given me a stuffed puppy to keep me company. I called him Bear. When Bear started talking to me in my thoughts, I knew I'd reached a new depth of hopelessness. What the heck? I'd nothing left to lose. So I started conversing with him.

Bear and I chatted about various things. One topic I clearly recall was his lecture to me about the importance of playing and of taking time off from work to do that. In fact, that was the true definition of self-discipline: doing what your highest Self really and truly wanted. Right now, I could only imagine myself playing. I thought of the wooden train tracks hiding in our closet at home. In my thoughts, I pretended Bear and I were constructing the tracks and running the trains.

Bear was a source of great comfort.

In time, I was able to identify the one who was really conversing with me. It was my old friend Rebazar Tarz.

Rebazar stayed by my side constantly throughout the remainder of my hospital experience. He would be there in the corner of my eye when hospital staff were in the room or in front of me if I wanted to look right at him. Sometimes I found him in my dreams.

In one dream, we were riding a train in the mountains and sitting in the caboose.

"I don't mind riding in the back," I said, finding a cushion to sit on.

"The goal is to sit in the conductor's seat," Rebazar informed me. "This healing journey will be over when you sit in the front."

Every day, I tried to imagine myself walking toward the front of the train. However, I never seemed to be able to leave the caboose.

I began to dream regularly about riding this train through the mountains. When the train was headed into a tunnel, it was a warning of new challenges ahead. When the train was ready to exit a tunnel, I knew things would get better for me in my hospital life.

Each day I would check inwardly to see where my train was and where it was headed. One morning I noticed a particularly dark tunnel approaching. "Oh boy, now what?" I thought.

"We've lowered your intravenous lidocaine," my cardiologist announced when he visited that afternoon. The tone of his voice suggested he thought this was very good news. "It's time to wean you off it, so you can go home."

"Go home?" I couldn't do that! My heart was too weak. I became fearful, and my heart promptly fell into v-tach.

Two nurses rushed in. One gave me a shot of lidocaine to stop the arrhythmia. The other returned my intravenous dose to its previous amount.

Once my heart rate normalized, the dish-rag-like feeling returned. I was too exhausted to move a muscle.

My doctor was not happy with me. "The next time I come in," he said sternly, "I will again broach the subject of you going home, and you will keep your heart rate normal."

I had three days to become mentally okay with going home.

So I practiced thinking about it. I'd let my mind wander back to my house for a moment, and then for two moments, and for longer and longer stretches of time. I wanted to be comfortable with the idea that whatever happened, I would be okay. Of course, I KNEW that whatever happened, I would be okay, and yet until that knowing drifted into my mind and settled there, I was a wreck thinking about it.

I knew I could not safely go home. If my heart failed again, and if the paramedics took twenty minutes to get to my house, and another twenty to get me to the hospital, I would not survive the ride. Going home was a death sentence. Furthermore, who would take care of me? Bob needed to work, my parents were unavailable to stay with me, and my brothers were both on military assignments overseas. We discussed live-in help, but that would empty my bank account within a few weeks.

The problem was, I had no place to go. I could not stay in the hospital. Nobody was available to take care of me, and I could not afford help. For the first time I felt what it was like to be a burden to family and society.

It would be better if I died.

Knowing what heaven was like, I was not afraid to go there again.

I wrote my problem onto a scrap of paper and asked God to take my life. I then crunched up the paper and threw it away.

This was my way of handing the problem over to a higher power.

The next morning I knew something had shifted, because when I awoke, my train was no longer in the tunnel. It was traveling along the edge of the mountain, in full sunlight.

My next angel arrived soon thereafter, in the form of a hospital social worker.

"We have good news," she said when she came to visit. "Your insurance company will pay for a stay at a rehabilitation center, where you can gain some strength before you go home."

I couldn't thank her enough.

Although I knew leaving the hospital was a bad idea, I trusted that this was my only possible step. I would wait another couple of days for the paperwork for my transfer to be completed.

By now I was able to take short walks up and down the hall and to watch television. One evening, I saw a documentary about a boy in Mexico who was born crippled. The boy was a gifted writer, whose poetry captured the heart of an American surgeon. The doctor agreed to give him reconstructive surgery that would allow him to walk.

The first time the boy got up from his wheelchair—the first step he ever took in his life—was a moment captured on film. To my incredible amazement, the boy held a drawing of one of the spiritual masters with whom I was familiar. His name is Lai Tsi.

I asked Bob for a copy of the same drawing, which we had at home. With this Mexican boy as my mentor, I held the picture of Lai Tsi as Bob wheeled me out of the comfort and safety of the hospital, into my next adventure in the rehab center.

Little did anyone know how soon I'd be back.

The nursing home was comfortable. The décor was homey, and I was free to walk around the facility, sit in the recreation room, or play with the resident cats—if I could find them. The staff were extremely busy and left me alone except for brief check-ins and to dispense meds. I shared a room with another woman, who was relearning how to speak after a stroke. So we were unable to hold a conversation.

My first night there, I laid awake trying to acclimate to my new environment. As quiet as it was—as wonderful as it felt to be free of the I.V. pole—I still felt restless. I thought about my near-death experience. Maybe I could funnel some of the peace I found in the inner worlds back into my presence circumstances?

I got far more than I expected.

I slipped out of my body and soared above a golden landscape. The currents swept me upward toward a temple with a rooftop of many rounded domes. I felt welcome here and approached the temple's massive doors. They opened. Inside, a forest of white marble columns supported the impossibly tall ceiling.

The Sound sang in my ears. In the core of my being, I knew the source of that music emanated from the center of this temple beyond the maze of marble. Reaching that source was my goal. But how to get there? There were thousands of pillars. Once past the first few, I was aware that I could easily get lost among them. Remaining found was part of the test.

Instinctively I sought the presence of Harold, my spiritual guide, who has never failed to help me in tight situations. He was there, somewhere to my right. I felt safe and encouraged.

He gave me a piece of advice: "The only way to keep from getting lost among the columns is to keep your ears tuned to the Sound."

He then communicated that this temple was a training ground. It was meant for those who had forgotten their purpose in life and wandered from their destiny.

I quickly learned that a wrong turn would dim the Sound and my heart would squeeze slightly. It would relax when I got back on track, and that sweet Sound would play again. This would be my mission—to stay in tune with that Sound. It was how I would survive in my outer life, too, and keep heading in the direction I was supposed to go. Here now, it was how I would successfully navigate the maze of marble.

I've heard people say "I'm in touch with the Light, now what?" Or "Now that I hear the Sound, is there anything more?" I had wondered about that too. Now the answer was mine.

Just watch. Just listen.

The more I listened, the deeper into my cells the Light and Sound was able to penetrate. When I felt completely inundated, I realized I had become the Sound. I floated on its river and then I was the river.

Suddenly, my movement through the columns felt perfectly timed and coordinated with all the rest of life. I was dancing with the Sound, and it was drawing me forward.

When I arrived at what I perceived to be the center of the temple, I stood face to face with a gently turning pillar of liquid golden light many stories tall.

Curiosity burned within me.

"You bring a piece of this with you."

The communication came from the Light itself. The invitation did not describe something about to happen, but the recounting of a factual event. I tasted its future—it was something I had yet to do. At the same time, it was something I was already doing, even though I had yet to capture the piece of the molten golden essence. And yet, the past was also involved, as I knew the task had already been accomplished.

It occurred to me that I must be beyond time in order to have this perception.

I used this awareness to figure out how to approach the Light and how to extract a bit of it, to fulfill the command. To do so, I simply remembered how it was that I had accomplished the task. A moment later, I held some in my hand.

Next, I found myself following orders that I could not clearly hear, and yet my path was somehow pre-ordained. I had the sensation of a steady movement downward, as though riding a down escalator, in what seemed to be a vehicle of structured light.

I was free to look around. What captured my attention was the golden light I held in my palm. It began to burn. I tossed it back and forth between my hands to ameliorate the fire. Dropping it was not an option. It didn't even occur to me that I might let it go.

The golden light grew smaller and cooler as we descended through a thick layer of clouds. The air grew heavier and I had to pay attention to my breathing until the extra labor became habitual. Soon the object in my hands became cold, clear, and white.

It felt precious. I held it up to look at it more closely. It was angular and gem-like. The ambient light of this world—still many times brighter than a sunny day on Earth—played with it. Prism-like, the gem separated the light into all seven colors of the rainbow. It also held the colors within itself.

I knew what I was looking at because I had seen one before many years ago. I was looking into a seven-color-ray-bearing Therapy Diamond.

The semi-conscious realization of what was happening shut off my memory of the rest of the experience. I had given up therapeutic diamonds and gemstones years ago and had no desire to study them again.

I wanted nothing to do with them.

From the sound of my roommate's breathing, I could tell she was sleeping.

I turned on the light and picked up a book that AriaRay had given me by Roald Dahl. Now all I wanted to do was escape from my inner reality and read about Matilda.

14

THE TROUBLE WITH DIAMONDS

*I*n 1987, David and I would regularly sit on the couch and meet with Hahn to find out which guardian we would learn from next. I would hold a tape recorder. We would begin by closing our eyes, singing HU, and then inviting Hahn to visit. He was always right there, as though waiting for us.

As he stepped into my body, I stepped out so not to get in his way. He used my eyes to see and my voice to speak with David. When he and David spoke, I always stood nearby listening and watching.

"You have a visitor," Hahn said one day.

A woman walked toward us, whom I recognized as the head of the Healing Council.

"The Guardian of Diamond," Hahn announced.

We had originally met in the Valley of the Crystal when the assignment with the gemstone guardians was given. I felt as though I'd known her all my life. Of all the guardians I had met, the Diamond Guardian was the brightest and most reminiscent of an angel. She was petite and slender, and the glow around her might be perceived as wings. She also emanated a glorious clarity of thought, which I enjoyed so much because it rubbed off on me for a short while after I was with her.

She was the only guardian who would not allow me to channel her, like the others did. Even if I invited her in, she would stay at a respectful distance, honoring the sanctity of my body and communicating with me nonetheless.

"Diamonds are a world apart from gemstones," she told us, "although they work well together therapeutically. Each gemstone carries a unique type of energy and each has its own special mission. Diamond's mission is to be the record-holder of all the frequencies in the universe, all the building blocks of creation."

She stood in front of me as she spoke, and I restated what she said so that David could hear.

"Each diamond crystal is like an encyclopedia. When a diamond crystal is cut, the encyclopedia opens to a page. Each page represents a different frequency or collection of them. With each new facet the diamond receives in the cutting process, a different page is revealed. Most of these pages represent frequencies that are supportive of the universe—but are not healthful to human beings. Faceting the diamond is the only way to reveal its color frequencies. When cutting is complete, most diamonds display frequencies other than colors. A rare few will present the seven color-ray frequencies. Fewer still will have a spectrum of color in a proper balance. These are the ones with therapeutic value."

"How are they therapeutic?" David asked. I did not have to repeat David's question because the Diamond Guardian could hear him. It was as though she was right there with us in the room.

"They have an affinity with the blueprints of optimal health and purpose housed within the highest levels of one's being. Blueprints define our true nature and our purpose in this lifetime."

"Are the DNA blueprints?"

"No. DNA molecules are not blueprints because they can be imperfect and can mutate. True blueprints represent the unspoiled ideal within us. DNA is part of our manifested matrix—meaning, what we've done with our blueprints.

"Blueprints and the manifested matrix are both sustained by spectrums. The journey to health involves transforming the spectrum of your manifested matrix into one that more closely matches that of your blueprints."

"So what exactly do Therapy Diamonds do?" David asked.

"Therapy Diamonds remind the body of its blueprints, which guide healing like the North Star once guided sailors in the night. Without its blueprints, an area that has been stressed might not know in which direction its healing should go. The tissue might mend, but underlying disharmony can remain. In trying to heal, the tissue might even take a path that strays away from the ideal.

"The proper use of Therapy Diamonds can produce deeply significant positive shifts in an individual's health and wellness. They clear the unwanted energies that fog and distort blueprint information. They awaken the blueprints, and help them advance their influence into your life. Therapy Diamonds feed the body with their color ray spectrums so you can better recognize your blueprints. And they reorganize the body into a liquid crystal, so that you can better receive the blueprint information.

"Blueprints guide atoms, molecules, organs, and systems, as well as the body, emotions, memory, mind, and intuition. You, as a being, have a blueprint that guides your purpose in life, too.

"Your unresolved troubles indicate a separation between yourself and your blueprints. The greater your troubles, the wider the separation. Therefore, the more closely your blueprint spectrum reflects itself in your life, the more closely you are following your life path. The same is true for any part of your body."

The potential of seven-color-ray-bearing Therapy Diamonds was truly exciting. Here was a tool that could remind the body of its truth. Because each individual's blueprint was so unique, nothing but a perfect mirror could accurately bring it forward. Therapy Diamonds could be that mirror.

I felt awed and inspired by the potential. What a gift Therapy Diamonds could be—especially to the leaders of our world!

The Diamond Guardian offered to teach me how to recognize them and I readily agreed. I had no clue what I was getting into.

For my initial lessons, the Diamond Guardian invited me into her world. We sat on marble benches at a round marble table in the center of a garden with geometrically shaped flower beds. The air was filled with the scent of roses that grew upon vines woven through the trellises that arched overhead. A crisp blue sky suspended two suns—one on each horizon—and a moon that was either closer or larger than our own. The beauty could have been distracting. I had to give my full attention to the guardian's instruction.

She sat at the table across from me and held a Therapy Diamond in her hands.

"In order for a diamond to be therapeutic," she said, "it must evenly and efficiently project its color rays throughout the body and aura. This is best accomplished by round diamonds, as opposed to squares or pears. While shape is important for Therapy Diamonds, clarity is critical.

"Without proper use, it is possible that a diamond's inclusions [the imperfections in a diamond's crystalline matrix] can be imprinted into a person's body and aura. They can cause significant energetic obstructions in the individual's energy flows and, worse, in their manifested matrix."

"Should a Therapy Diamond be flawless?"

"That would be impractical because few flawless diamonds exist."

She showed me what types of inclusions were okay, and gave me guidelines for their acceptable size and location.

"Purity is also important," the Diamond Guardian said. "A diamond that is completely colorless, physically speaking, is the most pure. It is comprised solely of carbon atoms. As other atoms enter the carbon matrix, or when the carbon matrix forms imperfectly, the diamond can take on physical color. The less physical color in a diamond, the more swiftly and directly the diamond's energetic color can bring forward blueprint information."

She handed me the diamond she was holding. It was as big as my thumbnail. Having had no previous experience with diamonds, I had no idea how unusual its size was. Later I learned this one must have weighed over ten carats.

"Now let's learn to see a diamond's energetic color."

She showed me how to hold the diamond in my palm, with its table, or upper flat surface, facing me.

"What do you see?" she asked.

The diamond's colors sparkled. "I see the color," I exclaimed. Could it be that easy?

"Describe what you see."

"The colors are like flashes, and they move when I move the diamond." I could identify all the colors in the rainbow.

"You are seeing the diamond's fire. This is a physical property—not its energetic spectrum. All nicely-cut round brilliant diamonds will display fire under certain lighting conditions." Then she said, "Look more deeply."

I noticed how the diamond's facets reflected light and dark and described this.

"This is the diamond's scintillation," she said. "Look more deeply."

I realized her suggestion to look deeply meant to look differently. I relaxed my gaze. I could feel myself move into a trance-like state.

The gardens in my peripheral vision disappeared, and my attention both narrowed and broadened at the same time. Finally, the faint glow of a spectrum seemed to appear inside and around the stone. The spectral colors grew bright and unmistakable.

"I see them!" I exclaimed, and of course, my lapse in attention caused the vision to disappear.

The Diamond Guardian smiled.

My next test would be to see the spectrum of physical diamonds.

David ordered a special microscope designed for viewing diamonds and made arrangements to receive a parcel of them. When they arrived, we met with the Diamond Guardian in our bedroom office.

"A Therapy Diamond has to meet strict physical and energetic parameters," she impressed upon us. "Foremost, it must carry a full spectrum of the seven color rays."

The Diamond Guardian showed me how to hold the diamond and led me into the trance-like state required to see the non-physical colors.

"Physical eyesight cannot tell the difference between a diamond that carries healing color rays and one that does not. Then again, physical eyesight cannot see frequencies period. Physical eyes see color rays only when a prism reveals them."

I looked at the diamond I was holding. I saw nothing. I tried looking at it from various depths of trance. I tried and tried again.

The Diamond Guardian was patient.

What was I doing wrong? Obviously, I wasn't getting it. Finally, I had to admit my failure. "I don't see a spectrum in this diamond."

"I don't either."

Really?

"Very few diamonds carry a spectrum."

I felt relieved.

We tried looking at another and then another.

"Don't hold that one," she warned. "It carries certain non-color-ray frequencies that can be harmful to the human body."

I set it down immediately and picked up another.

Eventually we found one that she liked.

"This one has the seven colors," she said. "Try to find them."

I considered her choice of words. She did not ask me to "see" the colors, but to "find" them. I learned I could not look directly at the diamond. I had to shift something within me, some manner of perception. I had to relax my vision, expand my scope of awareness, and allow my brain to receive and interpret what the diamond was showing me. I found the colors by adjusting my perception... and then I saw them. Plain as day.

"Notice how the seven colors are in relatively equal proportions. In this case—and if the physical parameters are also met—then we have a Therapy Diamond.

"If any one color dominates the spectrum, with all other colors in relatively equal proportions, then the diamond would be called by the dominant color, such as a 'Therapeutic Green Diamond' for a diamond whose spectrum was strongest in green."

Most of the diamonds I received for evaluation were non-therapeutic. Only a small fraction carried color rays. Then, not all of these carried the color rays in the proper proportions. Some spectrums would be "off" and others tainted with interfering frequencies. Some diamonds carried frequencies that would make me feel sick if I didn't recognize them soon enough and set them aside. Otherwise, I'd fall asleep or be knocked out of phase with myself and be unable to work for the remainder of the day.

I learned first-hand about a particularly insidious type of diamond whose energies produce a mirror-like quality that reflects thoughts. If I wanted to see a color-ray-bearing diamond—that's what would appear. So one of my tests of a true therapeutic diamond would be to try to imagine some object within it. If I tried to see a beautiful spectrum and saw it, and then tried to see a puppy or a pickle jar and that's what I saw, then that diamond would immediately go into the reject pile.

The trouble with this particular type of diamond was that if it was applied like a seven-color-ray Diamond, it could disassociate a person from her body. I've had this unlucky experience, and I don't like it at all. It felt as though parts of me were in my body and parts were elsewhere. It became impossible to think clearly or to connect thoughts with actions. To clear myself of this diamond's influence required using an authentic seven-color-ray Therapy Diamond to reset my blueprint connection.

"What about the diamond in my wedding ring?" I asked. "Will it hurt me if it isn't therapeutic?"

"Metal prongs act like a cage," she replied. "Diamonds mounted in metal cannot radiate their frequencies. Likewise, if your engagement ring happens to consist of a color-ray-bearing diamond, the mounting will cage its colors too. Therapy diamonds are applied loose and in special, very specific ways."

The Diamond Guardian taught us some of these ways.

As you can imagine, being the only one with the ability to declare which diamonds were therapeutic brought up a slew of conundrums. Tantamount was my own sense of integrity. Diamonds are expensive—especially those that have such pristine physical parameters. Because of the time-intensive labor involved in selecting the therapeutic ones, plus all the work involved in procuring, shipping, insuring, grading, organizing, and cataloging them, we sold them at a premium.

To select the diamonds, I had to be calm, centered, and at peace. Some days, I simply could not move myself into the state required to view them energetically. Because the parcels we would receive contained tens of thousands of dollars-worth of diamonds, the cutters who sent them to us were eager to get them back as soon as possible. This added to the pressure.

Another problem arose when other people thought they could identify therapeutic diamonds. I did not know this was happening until I saw a friend and customer of ours at a restaurant in Minneapolis. We were seated at a nearby table enjoying breakfast.

"There's something wrong with her aura," I said to David.

"What do you mean?" He looked over at our friend.

"I couldn't help but notice. It's an anomaly of such intensity that only a diamond could produce it."

He was concerned that something had gone wrong with the diamond we had sold to her. "How do you think it happened?"

"I have no idea."

"You should talk to her. Find out."

I leaned toward him and whispered, "I can't do that! I shouldn't be looking at people's auras!"

"As a rule you don't. But something caught your attention."

He was right. I fiddled with the food left on my plate and found another excuse. "I can't just go up to her and say, 'I think your diamond is hurting your energy field.' That is not appropriate."

"It is not appropriate to let her go on this way. You need to find out what she is doing wrong."

I deliberated. I wrestled with myself. I looked within for guidance.

I expected my inner guide to reprimand me for looking at someone's aura without their permission and tell me to mind my own business. Instead, I got an urge to get up and go talk to her. So I did.

We chatted awhile. Then I said "Are you still working with diamonds?"

She said she was.

"I'm sorry to interfere," I began to stumble over my words, "but I couldn't help notice that something doesn't look right in your energy field. I'm so sorry..."

She touched my arm and cut me off. "You don't need to say another word." She was so grateful that I had said something, and then admitted she had bought a supposed therapeutic diamond from someone else. Unfortunately, she had gotten the two diamonds confused and did not know which was which. She was wearing them both.

Back then, I taught people how to wear therapeutic diamonds by taping them to their body. Today I no longer recommend this practice. Too many diamonds had gotten lost by falling out of loosened placement tape.

We went to her hotel room and sorted out the therapeutic one from the imposter. I worked on her energy field with the true color-ray-bearing diamond to correct the anomalies that the other had created.

This was an incredibly humbling experience for me.

Another customer who was also buying imposter therapeutic diamonds reminded me of the saying about how the student inevitably surpasses the master. This comment was meant to justify the other seller's supposed expertise in determining a diamond's therapeutic value. However, this seller of diamonds had taken only one class with me. Nor had I ever taught her—nor anyone—my evaluation methods.

To my horror, I learned that this person was testing diamonds by holding them in her hand with the table of the diamond down. This meant that any harmful frequencies a diamond might be carrying were imparted into her body. It was a dangerous practice.

How briefly had knowledge of Therapy Diamonds been made public, and how quickly it had been abused!

When it comes to diamonds, I have seen inspiring acts of generosity. I have also seen the worst of greed, attachment, lust, anger, and vanity arise in otherwise spiritually devoted individuals. I truly doubted our society's readiness to learn about the healing uses of diamonds.

Working with Therapy Diamonds was a path defined by the sharpest of razors. I did not want to be tested—and fail. Despite the positive impact diamonds could have when used properly, their potential misuse did not seem worth the risk. It was easier to let the diamonds go and decide never to work with them again. And so I did.

15

ANOTHER MEETING WITH
THE DIAMOND GUARDIAN

Christmas 2004, and the nursing home where I was recuperating was festively decorated. I made it my duty to visit the other inmates (as I called us), to offer some company to those less mobile than I was.

Most instructive was the man down the hall in the extra-large single room with the polished wood floor and nice wall-paper. He was confined to his bed, alone and lonely. I shared with him the small bear and balloon someone had sent me for Christmas. I tied the balloon to his bedrail and he held the bear while we chatted. His well-dressed family took the gifts away when they came to visit him. While they were his, they cheered him up.

It was a stark reminder that wealth buys you neither health nor happiness—nor a loving family. I've always known this, but this was the first time I saw it firsthand. If my priorities weren't already set, this experience glued them into place. People are most important. Later on, when I began my gemstone business, I would make sure that people were always the priority.

I also visited the woman across the hall, whom I had become friendly with. She was fascinated by my near-death experience, and I enjoyed the relief she seemed to experience when I recounted the few details that I felt comfortable sharing.

My best Christmas gift was a visit from AriaRay and Kellan. We exchanged hugs and songs, and said goodbye all too quickly. I was gaining strength with the daily walking I was giving myself, and hoped to see my children again soon.

Monday, December 27, 2004, Bob had gone to visit his family, who lived about four hours away. I had encouraged him to go and had assured him that I was well taken care of and would not need him. The food at this facility was remarkably good, and I wolfed down breakfast when the call came for my first formal exercise session. I was not familiar with the schedule and did not want to be late. I hurried to brush my teeth and get ready, without realizing the rush was straining my heart more than it could bear.

I walked a little too swiftly to the exercise room, where exercise machines were neatly arranged along every wall. I saw my new friend from across the hall, and the attendant sat me down at a machine next to hers. He attached our forefingers to heart rate monitors. My friend and I chatted as we waited for the attendant to give us the go-ahead to start the exercise. I was in a good mood, feeling well, and looking forward to the rehab session.

Suddenly I began to feel funny and noticed the numerical readout on my heart rate monitor start to climb. Drugs were keeping my heart rate around 60 beats per minute. On the monitor, I could see it rising to 65 beats per minute, then 70, then 81.

"Uh oh," I said aloud.

"Are you okay?" my friend asked.

The monitor read 90, 95, and then BHAM!

I fell off my chair, crying out with each BHAM as the I.C.D. jolted me repeatedly. Between jolts, I calmly told my friend I'd been through this before and I'd be okay. Yet I must have been a sight, sprawled on the floor, my body jerking uncontrollably with every kick of the life-saving device.

The attendants quickly cleared everyone from the room, and a nurse called Bob, who returned home immediately.

My next angel was the paramedic who was able to pin an I.V. into my tiny, worn-out veins in his very first attempt.

It was another gift to be back in the hospital, albeit the emergency room. I was met by friends—doctors and nurses who knew me. They hooked up my I.C.D. to a computer and marveled at the printout. "Did it really fire thirty-two times?" a nurse asked incredulously.

I said I'd stopped counting at twelve.

I was in good hands, and the lidocaine was back in my veins.

*   *   *

As I recovered in the intensive care unit from the shocks of the I.C.D., my mind wandered to my near-death experience. It provided solace, hope, and reassurance.

I realized how the term "near-death experience" implies a brush with finality. Death is not final, just a transition into another life. So, although I might continue to use the term so that people know what I'm talking about, I think it's more accurate to say "heaven-life experience."

As I drifted in my memories, I recalled a detail of my heaven-life experience that I'd forgotten. One day when I was happily fulfilling my job of transcribing information I'd learned in temples in yet higher heavens, I was invited to a meeting of a group of light beings, dignified and splendid. I counted about a dozen. They were gathered around a long white conference table. I stood at the foot of it. This was the Healing Council I had met years before. Although they looked familiar, my conscious mind blocked the memory of their identity.

They had a message for me: "You will spend a lifetime recording everything you've learned here."

I understood that they were talking about the lifetime I was living in then—in heaven. Years later I would realize what they really meant. They were talking about my work with Gemstone Therapy. The information I was bringing down from above was about the therapeutic use of gemstones and diamonds.

A nurse's aide came in to check my vital signs. I pretended I was asleep to avoid unnecessary conversation. I felt frustrated by the interruption. When she left, I covered my eyes with my pillow to pretend I was anywhere other than the I.C.U. Soon, the darkness drew me into itself. My attention moved back to the meeting with the Healing Council. No longer was this a memory. My experience with them had moved into present time and became very real.

In the inner worlds, the woman seated at the head of the table stood up and invited me to go for a walk. She was petite and slender, and her long hair glistened. I had blocked the memory of her identity too.

We walked down a short hallway and entered a greenhouse filled with flowering plants. Their perfume scented the air. To my wonderment, the large domed room was alive with thousands of colorful butterflies. I had never seen anything like this before and was completely enthralled. The butterflies flitted about from one flower to the next, sometimes landing on our heads or arms.

We sat on a bench carved of colorful jasper beside a hedge abounding with red and pink hibiscus.

"I've heard you are interested in the life-giving color rays," she said.

"Very much."

"Color rays originate in the white light. Sunlight carries all seven rays, and yet they cannot be seen by physical eyes except when separated by a prism. So people do not realize how directly colors support life.

"The cosmos is another source of color rays. They are strewn about the universe in vast swaths of random spectrums produced by certain cataclysmic stellar events. Other fields of cosmic color are intentionally placed in space. They are the legacy of ancient beings of unfathomable intelligence who laid them there to spur evolution. As a solar system passes through these great wandering drifts of color, evolution is stimulated. People experience an outpouring of ideas and enhanced creativity. History is marked by the leaps of forward momentum made possible by these cosmic rendezvous."

"Can we avoid them?"

"Who would want to?" she shrugged. "These color rays rain upon us freely and ultimately lead to greater enlightenment."

She picked a hibiscus and held it to her nose. "We can also receive color rays from nature—especially when our hearts are open to them. My body easily recognizes the red in this hibiscus. The flower is a living thing. It is able to strengthen my ability to call in more red ray."

"A silk flower wouldn't do that?"

"The life-energy of the living flower makes the difference."

She tucked the flower behind her ear. "Another source of color rays is within one's own self, from the inner bodies. These bodies are also unseen by physical eyes. Yet we know they exist by the feelings we get from our emotional body, the memories and sense of time and space afforded by our causal body and the thoughts that spring from our mental body. The inner bodies can be seen by the clairvoyant as layers of the aura and physically palpated by those dedicated to learning how."

I picked a flower of my own and twirled it while we spoke. "I don't understand how the subtle bodies relate to the aura. Are they the same?"

"In the three dimensions of the physical world, the emotional body has a larger energetic imprint than the physical body. So it appears like a layer of the aura extending beyond the physical body. The causal and mental bodies occupy even larger spaces in three dimensions, and so they appear as layers that reach beyond the emotional layer."

She was interrupted by a butterfly that landed on her nose. We both giggled. She lifted a finger in front of it and it hopped on.

"Yes, love is also a source of color rays," she said as though speaking to the butterfly, which then flitted onto a nearby flower.

"In a healthy person, color rays circulate from the subtle bodies to the physical body and back. Their movement is cleansing and renewing. As spectrums flow into the physical body, they feed and nourish it. Upon the return flow, the dross that the color rays have picked up dissipates into the universe.

"Color rays coming from the subtle bodies to the physical should be pure and life-giving. Positive thoughts and emotions are associated with pure color spectrums. Negative thoughts, words, and emotions will muddy the colors and feed us with less-than-ideal color nourishment—or none at all.

"When a person's spectrums radiate harmonious color rays, we inwardly perceive the individual as a good person. If we sense distrust or negativity in a person, it's due to the muddiness in that person's aura. It serves as a warning to other living beings that negativity is forthcoming."

I tried to sense what I was feeling from this woman's aura. The color spectrums were intense and bright. I felt overwhelmed. "Focus on what she's saying," I told myself. Otherwise I might lose the experience.

"Are you familiar with the chakras?" she asked me.

"Yes. The body has seven, along the front midline. I understand they bring energy into the body."

"That's right. Color rays from the sun, cosmos, and aura enter the body through the chakras. Healthy chakras distribute color rays wherever they are needed. They also dispel spent energies, like the lungs exhale carbon dioxide."

"What about the food we eat?" I asked. "Are they a source of color rays?"

She paused for a moment, as though considering how to answer the question.

"The reason why people can be meat-eaters, vegetarians, vegans, or fruitarians is a matter of color. It is not necessarily the physical nutrients these foods provide. The meat-eater's body is capable of extracting and converting the life energy of meat into color rays, while the vegetarian cannot. Likewise, some people can exist on fruit alone, because their bodies can convert fruit into full spectrums of color, while a meat-eater cannot.

"The bright, well-defined colors of fresh fruits and vegetables announce the life-energy in the food. Ingest this food and its atoms will nourish you with color rays—provided your cells can accept them. If the cells cannot, then your body will have to transform the food's life energy into a spectrum your body can recognize.

"If you eat food whose life-energy has been diminished or altered, then your body must work harder to convert the food's atoms into color-ray-bearing atoms. To do this, your body must lend the food color rays. If this awakens inherent color in the life-energy in the food, then the investment pays off. The food will return the life-energy loaned, plus more.

"If your body is unable to make this conversion, and you eat colorless food too often, your body will become depleted from the task of trying to wring color from the food."

I wondered, "Is excess fat a storehouse of color?"

"If your body is unable to derive color rays from a food, your body won't be able to receive its life energy. Food from which the body cannot derive life-giving energy tends to be stored as fat or to pass through undigested. Fatty tissue also contains accumulations of non-color-ray-bearing energies. These can come from non-nutritive additives included in processed food, foods whose energies the body does not recognize, as well as foods which are sometimes called 'empty calories.' These foods carry non-color-ray frequencies. The body has no idea what to do with non-color-ray frequencies, and so it stores them. Some non-color-ray-frequencies are stored in various places, such as on artery walls, in the brain, in the liver, or in the joints. Most are stored as fatty tissue."

I heard some commotion in the hallway, and remembered that my physical body was in a hospital bed. It sounded as though another patient needed immediate assistance. I turned on my side and carefully repositioned the arm that had the I.V. tube attached. I put the pillow back over my head to drown out the noise outside my room.

Fortunately, I was able to return easily to the inner-world green house. All I had to do was think about those beautiful butterflies, and my attention transported me back.

My friend was waiting for me. I knew she had more to share, and I was right.

"There's another source of color rays I want to remind you about," she said. "This source allows you to direct any color to any area of your body you choose. This is important because color rays can be used for healing. You can use them to evaluate and adjust the resident spectrum associated with any issue or condition, to correct color-ray imbalances, and to replace non-color-ray frequencies in the body with life-giving color rays.

"This source of color rays comes from the Earth herself. Earth is special because it is a storehouse of color rays that support life. In this way, the Earth is self-sustaining. It is why so many species flourish there. Earth's ability to produce life-energy involves her living core, her atmosphere, her water, and her crystals.

"Earth is a vast resource of crystals, both in quantity and diversity. Certain ones are color-ray bearing. When they are fashioned into gemstone spheres and worn, they offer color rays in concentrated form. This is especially helpful for correcting deficiencies in life-energy and ameliorating ailments that can arise as a result."

Wait.

Pardon my stubbornness. I still did not want to hear about gemstones nor the crystals they came from.

Fortunately, I got distracted by my cardiologist, who had come for a visit.

My cardiologist had already earned his angel wings in my eyes. He proved himself once again when he said it was time to get me on the heart transplant list. It was a big step for him.

"I've never lost a patient to transplant," he confessed. He had been able to save his patients' hearts with good doctoring alone.

"It's my destiny," I tried to explain. I told him that when the ambulance took me from my house, I intuitively knew I would not be coming home without a new heart. I thanked him for all he had done and was at peace with what seemed to be the next logical step. I was ready to get onto the waiting list.

For whatever reason, my insurance company would not pay for a heart transplant at this hospital. The nearest hospital they would accept was in another city. Because I might not live through the ambulance ride, I would be transported by helicopter.

Before I left, I had one last visit from the electrophysiologist cardiologist in charge of my I.C.D. To my surprise, he let me give him a respectful embrace.

I told him I'd made up a rhyme: "I will survive in 2005."

16

CONVERSATIONS WITH MY ORGANS

The new hospital took some getting used to. It was in a bigger city, so the rooms were smaller and the view out the window was simply another building. This felt claustrophobic until I learned to make it feel cozy.

I expected to get on the heart transplant list right away. Not so. They said my health needed to improve first.

So I considered what I could do to heal myself.

I'd heard of a technique in which you imagine white light streaming down from above, entering your head, and filling your entire body. I gave it a try. The Light that remained with me since the near-death experience was everywhere, surrounding me and penetrating me. I could not imagine it being separate from myself and outside my body. Therefore I could not imagine it coming into my body.

I also tried sound techniques, such as singing mantra, specifically the HU. Most of the time, I didn't have the energy to sing aloud, so I imagined listening to someone singing HU. Sometimes I would listen to different organs in my body sing this sound.

The HU is a powerful mantra. It is fully charged with the love of God. When I sing it or listen to it, as a long drawn out sound, it uplifts, purifies, and opens my heart to a greater inflow of Spirit. This can bring about changes, such as healing. While I listened to the HU in my imagination, I would consciously surrender to any changes that might come about, whatever they might be. I would let the Sound have its way.

It was during one of these HU thinking sessions that I got the idea to talk with my organs and cells, to prepare them for the inevitable transplant. The idea met resistance on both sides: I was afraid to hear what my organs and cells might say, and I think they were afraid of what I might tell them, too.

So I started with my toes. After all, how consequential would they be in the upcoming surgery?

"Hello, toes," I said, and wriggled them.

They did not reply right away. I sensed they heard me and were ignoring me.

Then their telepathic reprimand was clear: "You've lived with us for forty-four years without noticing us—except to cover us with toenail polish. You've never said hello or thanked us for helping you walk."

Wow. I had taken them for granted. I apologized and gave them a little massage with hospital lotion.

"I really do appreciate you, toes. I know you help me to stand upright. Let's think of all the places you have helped me go." I thought about beaches, mountain trails, and the aisles of health-food stores. "I really am grateful to you."

They forgave me.

I wondered if we would ever be able to walk in any of those favorite places again.

This spurred an idea to make a formal announcement to all my organs and cells. "Hey gals, we need to work together to get well enough to get on the heart transplant list so that we can be completely healthy once again."

I felt a lot of resistance this time.

"You can't just barge into our world and tell us what to do," I heard Liver say.

"You're part of my body."

"You are a part of ours too," the organs said as one voice. This put me in my place. "You are no more important than we are," they said. "You can't live without us. We can't live without you. We think that makes us a team."

That made sense. "Aren't I in charge?"

Silence.

"Well then who is?"

"Heart is in charge of the body. You are in charge of our entire being, our well-being, and our destiny. You're the one who decides a life purpose, and we in turn allow you to fulfill that purpose."

"And who are you?"

"I'm the Spirit of your Liver. I'm second in command, and you have a lot to learn."

Wow. I felt humbled. "I'm listening," I said respectfully.

"Each organ has its own intelligence center, or spirit, and we deserve some respect. It was rude to tell us we needed to work together to get on the heart transplant list. Maybe we don't want to get a new heart."

"Oh?"

Obviously the intelligence centers of the organs each had a conscious individuality. They had a voice and liked having it heard. They had insights and information that I wasn't consciously aware of, and they had feelings, too.

I realized I could not just barge into my organs' world and demand they make changes. They needed to get to know me first. We needed to develop a relationship. In the process, I would learn about them, and the community of organs they lived among and how their actions influenced each other.

Learning how to converse with the spirits of my organs would eventually play a big role in my future work with my Gemstone Therapy clients. It was just as easy to talk with the spirits of other peoples' organs as it was my own.

In my conversations with my organs, I learned that some parts of me were genuinely afraid of another open-heart surgery. They were suspicious of a new heart and the process of getting one.

In one conversation my heart said, "I'm sorry for the trouble I'm causing. I'm sorry for putting everyone through such misery." She was okay to transfer her authority to a new heart. "I promise to leave as gracefully as possible."

"You are wonderful still," Stomach told her.

"You're doing your best," Feet said.

"You are loved no matter what," Lungs said.

One after another, other organs gave solace to Heart.

"I want all of you to live," Heart said.

After a pause, Lungs assured everyone, "We can survive the transplant and the surgery. I've been on the heart-lung machine before. It was hard to let go control and harder to take it back, but we did it. And we can do it again."

"We have the strength to do it," Legs promised. "We may be weakened, but we have enough stored resources to see us through."

"Do we have enough time to say good-bye?" Stomach asked. "I want to express my gratitude,"

"The transplant isn't happening now," Lungs said.

"We don't know when the transplant will happen," I said. "We're not even on the waiting list."

Anyone reading this who thinks I was imagining these conversations might be right. Maybe I was. Yet the gratitude and sincerity I felt coming from my organs felt genuine and often brought me to tears. The welling up of joy within me as a result of these communications was strong medicine.

It was also sobering. Most of my organs did not believe that transplant would be a winning ticket to health. My body knew the truth better than I did. In my telepathic communications with my parts, I learned that the heart transplant would be but a step on my journey to greater health.

What did my cells think? Rather than speak to billions of them individually, I learned the cells can communicate in a common voice. Speaking to my cells was like speaking to a separate organ. I could do the same with the collective intelligence of my molecules and atoms, as well.

"We believe a new heart would make us all feel a lot better," the Spirit of the Cells said.

Most of my organ spirits agreed.

With little else to do in the hospital, I had plenty of time to chat with every part of my anatomy individually, and eventually did so.

* * *

Waiting to get on a waiting list felt like treading water. I was headed nowhere. It also gave me an odd sense of freedom. Once I got on the list, it meant that at any moment, a doctor could walk in and tell me that in five or six hours, I'd be having major heart surgery.

I might live through the surgery. Or I might not.

When I was only waiting to wait, I didn't have to worry about my life being so rudely interrupted. I felt safely quarantined from such surprises. It was an odd respite from the inevitable.

Ten days after being admitted to the new hospital, my health had improved to the point that I was ready to wait for real. They officially put me on the heart transplant waiting list. As the days passed and no call came, I began to understand what waiting meant. If you want something to happen—especially something that will change your life—then waiting for it can drive you nuts. It can lead to impatience, anxiety, depression, and desperation. I had my turn with each.

One day, Bob told me he'd met a woman in the hospital lobby whose husband had been there for over a year and was still waiting for his heart. The news was humbling. I could be waiting for a very long time.

I had to stop waiting and start living.

I declared my hospital room a healing temple. Every morning I would uplift the room's vibrations in some small way. I'd prune the dead leaves and petals from the flowers and plants that friends had generously sent, and dust the window-sill they sat on.

I started a collage of get-well cards I had received. I tacked them on my room's bulletin board, and every few days would rearrange them, adding new ones, and placing others among the flowers on my window sill.

After a while, I had received so many cards that I kept the extras in a stack, wrapped in a ribbon that had once adorned a bouquet. I called them my Love Pile. They were a source of tremendous support, and I would read through them whenever I was feeling down. I have kept all the cards, even to this day.

I also decided to work on a novel I'd started in 1994 (*The Capstone Decision*, which I eventually self-published in 2009). Every day I took time to write—longhand. I looked forward to Bob's next visit when he would bring a laptop that my friends Brad and Diane offered to loan me.

In addition to the work I gave myself to do, I was visited by a steady stream of doctors, fellows, nurses, aides, phlebotomists, social workers, transplant coordinators, a psychiatrist, a clergywoman, and others. Physical therapists came three times a week to keep me exercising, and I did feel as though I was growing stronger.

It was always a joy when friends came to visit. I received some one-timers, and I had my regulars: Andy, Fred, and Randy, who always brought my standard requests of soft tissues, oranges, and avocados. Andy and Randy brought me a meal of gourmet raw foods for my birthday, which I coveted. I welcomed whatever fresh or homemade food anyone wanted to bring.

One day Fred brought in a kaleidoscope, compliments of his wife, Setsko. I'd gaze into it for long periods of time, marveling at its changing colors. One night, I held the kaleidoscope against the green and yellow lights on the side panels of my bed. The colors seemed to come alive, and I was transported back to the Great Library, where I had worked during my near-death experience.

The memories of writing at the big wooden table came alive. I noticed the words that poured upon the pages were a language I did not recognize. I spoke English, didn't I? But that was in a faraway time in what seemed like a distant incarnation. I was living in heaven now, my body had succumbed to a fatal arrhythmia, what seemed like a very long time ago.

I wondered about this language that I now transcribed.

"The cursive you use is the written language of the mind. It's a telepathic script, recognized and taught throughout the galaxies and worlds."

"Who said that?" I asked.

I looked around at the twenty-foot-tall stacks of books, beneath the impossibly high ceiling. The source of the voice was the angel I had met before, with the sparkles in her hair. She had been standing behind me.

"When you are ready," she said, sitting herself gracefully into a chair next to mine. "You will come back to find this script and know what you are reading. So will others. You are leaving a legacy for all."

I looked at what I was writing with new appreciation. These were not my words. They were someone else's work, something I had found in a higher level of heaven and transcribed here. I read what I had just written, and because conversation happens telepathically in heaven, it was as though I spoke aloud:

The Light and Sound forms waves, which I perceive as ribbons. A single ribbon represents the spectrum of a single atom.

Looking deeper, I notice the Sound binds the colors into a spectrum. At the same time, the spectrums translate the Sound from something cosmic and un-hearable to something that can be heard. The Sound unifies and organizes the Light, and the Light manifests the Sound.

The Light sings. The Sound plays. Together they enable life. Light and Sound is life.

"I wonder who the original author was?" I mused.

The angel gave me a warm smile and I knew: It had been her.

"Color rays are the secret of life," she said. "When something is imbued with a color ray spectrum, it is then capable of being a vehicle for conscious expression. It is therefore alive.

"The world is teeming with life: from the macro-beings who manifest as people, plants, and animals, to the micro-beings of the mineral, cellular, molecular, and atomic realms. There are also the cosmic beings: the planets, stars, and galaxies that house a singular intelligence similar to that of any human. Life abounds at all levels of manifestation—in all places and in all realms—and all have intelligence.

"Each intelligence is fed and sustained by a color-ray spectrum. Each houses consciousness."

I thought about the objects in my hospital room. Did they contain spectrums? The furniture: once living wood. The plastic tube of hand cream on my bed stand: the plastic made of petro-chemicals that were once living forests, crushed beneath weight and time. The paper in my books: also once-alive trees. The components of the television set: mostly plastics, metals, and glass. In time—perhaps a long time—they will break down into their elemental constituents and those elements will feed a life form. If they become a part of that life form and take on a color ray spectrum, then they too will be alive.

"All things either are alive, once-alive, or will one day support a life form."

The angel spoke the words that I had already transcribed in the great book. I looked into the pages and continued to read:

> No atom can be denied the experience of life. All will become involved in the expression of a Light and Sound spectrum, perhaps for a moment or maybe for a millennium.
>
> Color rays are Light and Sound and evoke consciousness. What is consciousness? It's easier to answer what it does. Consciousness sparks the potentially-living into the state of present-time-aliveness. It organizes and collects non-color-bearing atoms and molecules, and, following inherent blueprints, forms them into a vehicle that can express life energy and be a vehicle for color spectrums.

I stopped reading. It was more interesting to hear the words from the author herself. I gave the angel sitting beside me my full attention.

"As a human being, you have earned the right to captain a huge collection of living spectrums. They form your body, your emotions, your memories, and your thoughts. Being in charge of so many spectrums does not make your consciousness any better or higher. It does make your responsibility greater."

She leaned her elbows on the table and moved her hands as she spoke. "Life demands spectrums. Colors do not exist by themselves in nature. They are joined together in spectrums that consist of all seven colors of the rainbow.

"Dissect the atom and each subatomic particle will also carry a color-ray spectrum—as long as it supports a living being. Remove the life, and you remove the color rays. Remove the atom from the living body, and the atom will lose its colors.

"When a person nears death, it seems as though her color rays start to recede and become weakened. That is only the body's perspective. As the color rays recede from physical reality, they pool at a higher vibration. They form a capable and welcoming matrix for the Soul when it leaves the body."

I wondered if the angel knew about my donor. Were her color rays now beginning to recede? Did my donor know on some level this was happening? Could she feel it?

The angel continued, "This matrix of color ray spectrums that houses a Soul after death will revitalize and heal the remnants of any affliction experienced just before the death occurred. Sometimes a Soul is taken to a special healing temple to fully recover from the fatal illness or injury once suffered. This healing is a process of correcting the imbalances in the color ray spectrums involved.

"Colors support life. Color is life," she emphasized.

"Breathe in the atoms of air and they will remain colorless in your lungs until your body converts them to color-bearing, life-giving atoms. Though colorless atoms can oxygenate your body, only color-bearing ones will give it life. Only color-ray-bearing atoms constitute living tissue. Only color-ray-bearing atoms can heal.

"One way to increase the amount of color rays your body is able to receive is by drinking water."

"Water? Did I hear you correctly?"

"Yes. Water molecules in the sky form a prism that reveals the rainbow. Atmospheric water separates the sun's white light into colors. Likewise, the water in your body acts like a living prism. The body must be adequately hydrated for the prism-effect to occur. You need to drink fresh water and assimilate it in order for it to separate the life force inherent within your food into living color rays that your body can use.

"You can also increase the amount of color in your body by wearing color-ray-bearing gemstones."

I almost balked at the mention of gemstones. I had already done so twice because I thought that this chapter of my life was over for good. It wasn't polite to leave the conversation once again. Dutifully, and as neutrally as possible, I continued to listen.

"Seven gemstones are known specifically as color-ray bearing gemstones. These are Ruby, Carnelian, Yellow Sapphire, Emerald, Blue Sapphire, Indigo, and Amethyst. What sets these gemstones apart from other gems of color is that they carry a certain formula.

"The formula consists of light, in the form of the color ray each carries, and sound in the form of instructions. The instructions are like a script that teaches the body to convert non-color-ray bearing atoms and molecules into spectrum-bearing, life-giving atoms and molecules. Furthermore, if a gem carries your main color ray, then it can help your body call in all the color rays.

"The body needs color rays to live.

"Color is life."

She paused after each sentence for emphasis. "You will come to appreciate color," she predicted.

In the days to come, I would learn how right she was.

17

PHANTOM PAIN AND ECHOES

*R*ebazar Tarz was constant company. He appeared in his light body and usually sat on the windowsill to my right or stood beside it. I was able to see him almost as clearly as anything else—although he was always easier to see with my eyes closed. I thought it interesting that once I found him dozing. Even the masters must rest.

One morning, he boarded my inner-world train and invited me to join him. It was time for my next adventure through a tunnel. I did not brace myself for it, nor get worried or anxious. The tunnel was a fact. I would enter it and I would face the inevitable. So my day continued as usual, with me being only casually curious what would happen. Secretly, I hoped it meant I'd be called for transplant.

Late that afternoon, pain tore through my abdomen.

I gripped my nurse's leg as I bent over in agony. I knew it was a gallbladder attack because my gallbladder had been bothering me for several weeks. In fact, I think it had been acting up since childhood. Doctors at the previous hospital had already run a battery of tests. The doctors here had performed their own. I hoped this killer attack was the final evidence they needed to do something besides testing.

They did.

They took me off the transplant list.

My cardiologists told me I needed my gall bladder removed. If all went well, they said, I'd be back on the list in a few weeks.

A few weeks?

A day later one of my cardiologists told me that the doctoral fellow in charge of me arranged the surgery in record time. "He moved mountains for you," she said and marveled at the miracle. I'd be getting my gall bladder removed the following day. If all went well, I could be back on the list in ten days.

My doctor visited me again as they were rolling me into the operating room. "Gallbladder removal is a piece of cake," she assured me.

Not exactly. I felt very sick afterward. My next angel was Andy, who was there to hold my hand when I came back from the recovery room. It meant so much to me to have someone present, even as I drifted in and out of sleep.

Did I tell you that Bob was home with the flu? It would be a total of eighteen days that he wouldn't be able to visit me. They didn't want me to catch a cold. If I did, I couldn't be on the transplant list.

I was in reverse quarantine. That meant that anyone who wanted to enter my room had to put on a surgical mask and robe—even for the brief seconds it took the kitchen staff to put the food tray on my table. Every doctor, every nurse, everyone. Some took the precaution more seriously than others. I didn't say anything. I wasn't worried about catching a cold.

I was worried about having been taken off the transplant list for the gallbladder surgery. Would I miss my opportunity for a new heart? Even after I felt fully recovered, the doctors wanted to give me more time before putting me back on the list.

"Heart transplant is a huge thing," a doctor said. "You have to be strong enough."

Then Rebazar communicated something telepathically: I was comforted to learn that the individual who was destined to give me her heart was not yet ready to pass. The time period in which I was off the transplant list was necessary for my health. I would not miss my opportunity.

Two days after my gallbladder was removed, I awoke one morning to a familiar stabbing pain in my right side. If it wasn't for the four small scars on my belly proving to me that the gall-bladder was gone, I would have suspected another attack.

I said something to a nurse. Her reaction: "You don't have a gallbladder, so it can't hurt," made me realize I'd better keep quiet. Something was going on that the medical community could not understand.

I suspected that my body was holding stress from the surgery. I tried to relax, but the pain wouldn't let me. I called Kim, my craniosacral therapist, and told her about it. Did she have a suggestion for how I could unwind the pain myself?

She didn't think that was the problem. "You're experiencing phantom pain," she said.

While the physical organ had been removed, its energetic counterpart was still sick, and it was letting me know that in no uncertain terms.

"Maybe the gallbladder counterpart in your aura doesn't realize the physical organ is gone," Kim suggested.

After my morning rituals and the first wave of medical visitors had come by, I had some free time to get quiet. I got back into bed, closed my eyes, and focused on the pain.

"Body, do you know the source of this pain?" I asked. I could feel my intelligence centers scanning my insides.

"It isn't physical," came the reply.

147

That is what I suspected.

Gently, I stroked the painful area. Meanwhile, I focused on where my gallbladder once was, imagining what the landscape of my anatomy looked like without it. It seemed the surrounding tissues had filled in the gap, so it wasn't like an empty hole existed there—at least not physically.

Like tuning a radio dial to another station, I adjusted my inner vision to a higher vibration—that of the supraphysical plane. Looking at the area from this vantage point, I could see that the gallbladder looked swollen and inflamed. I could sense it was struggling with something, and fighting against itself. Was it trying to pass a phantom gallstone?

"Spirit of Gallbladder?" I called gently and non-verbally.

Like a compass needle finding north, the spirit aligned itself with the source of my voice. I called its name again. It seemed to be waking up from a long sleep. I knew it could hear me.

"Look around you," I said.

Its attention scanned its surroundings and noticed its physical counterpart was missing. "What happened?" it said glumly.

"Physical Gallbladder was removed."

I sensed it needed time to process this statement. Spirit of Gallbladder seemed so lost. "Now what?" it said. It sounded a little frightened, too.

"Now you no longer have to reflect pain and struggle," I replied.

More processing.

I felt the presence of someone approach. It looked like a guardian angel no taller than the length of my arm from elbow to wrist. She was a swirling mass of wispy light, with a face I could barely discern. I believe she was an angel for organs and she was focusing on Spirit of Gallbladder.

"It's time to go," she told it.

Physically I could feel the roots of my gallbladder's energetic counterpart loosen and lift from out of my side. The pain lessened. The angel's swirling light encompassed my gallbladder's energies, like wings wrapping around it.

"It's time to go," she repeated and lifted the gallbladder spirit from my body into the heavens above.

"Thank you Gallbladder," I said and filled myself with genuine gratitude for all the service my gallbladder had given me.

I would like to say that this ended the pain for good. Not so. I had still to learn about echoes. These are the responses of tissues to imprinted patterns. Even though all the sources of pain may be gone as well as the organs involved, the experience of pain digs deep grooves in the fabric of our being. The experience of echoes occurs as our body tries to iron out these grooves. It's a healing process, although it does not feel that way.

Fortunately, the next few times I felt a gallbladder attack the pain was progressively less. I knew the attacks were echoes. To promote healing, I imagined smoothing the wrinkles and grooves in the area—particularly at the causal aspect of my being. I've already mentioned the supraphysical, which I perceive as the energetic layer immediately above the physical body. Then there's the emotional body, which holds the feelings involved. The causal body holds the patterns I'm talking about. Then the mental body holds the attitudes, opinions, and beliefs that contributed to a condition.

In the case of my gallbladder, emotions were not the biggest issue. I was feeling the imprint of repetitive pain, which had affected my causal layer by creating patterns of pain and hence the echoes.

Perhaps I should say more about the causal body. While people can relate easily to the emotions and thoughts of the emotional and mental body, the causal body is somewhat foreign, although the concept of patterns repeating themselves is not an uncommon experience. Besides storing patterns, the causal body helps us perceive space and time. While the Spiritual Self perceives here and now, the causal body is responsible for determining there and then. Our sense of time and space is a causal-body construct. Our movement in space, from one place to another—even from one room to another—is a perception of causal awareness.

Our highest Spiritual Self sees our entire physical existence outside of time. In contrast, the causal intelligence sees the individual experiences as letters and sorts them into words that go in a certain order to form a sentence. It organizes experiences along a time track, dividing past from present and future. This allows our mind to perceive our life unfolding linearly. Experiences can then be better comprehended for the purpose of learning from them.

When it's hard to let go of a memory, or a pattern or an echo, it's often because our instincts tell us the associated experience taught us something so important that if we let go the memory the wisdom gained will be lost. So the body holds onto the memories long after their lessons have been learned. We carry the memories along, adding to our body's burden, rather than storing them in the causal body where they belong.

Wisdom gained always remains. Lessons learned become indelibly imprinted in our fabric. They become a part and essence of who we are. They become the voice of common sense, gut sense, and intuition. Then, of course, the next lesson is to pay attention. If we don't trust ourselves to listen to the wisdom gained, then the body is more likely to hold onto the old memories. They are insistent reminders.

A well-organized causal body consists of innumerable storage compartments neatly arranged according to time and space. In other words, experiences are stored based on when and where they occurred. Storage cells can be open or closed. When closed, the memories have served a purpose. They have contributed wisdom to our fabric, making us better human beings.

Storage units that remain open allow their contents to be readily accessible by the mind, emotions, and conscious recall. Units that should remain open contain records of experiences that would be in our best interest to remember: people's names, important conversations, and where we left the car keys. Storage cells that should be shut contain memories of traumatic experiences that haunt us and limit our ability to live healthy, fruitful lives.

We have the ability to open and close these storage units. After all, they're ours.

I've also learned that the causal body is a source of our beliefs because beliefs tend to be based on past experiences. Beliefs play a huge part in what we are able to manifest and enjoy in our life. It is a false, limiting belief that we cannot control our thoughts, memories, and emotions. I have learned that it is a false and limiting belief that we cannot change our beliefs.

Back in the hospital, I recognized this and wondered what limiting beliefs might be preventing me from getting a new heart. For one: Did I believe I was worthy to receive one?

18

INNER PREPARATIONS

*F*eeling unworthy to receive a new heart is a common challenge for people waiting on the transplant list. I didn't believe this issue haunted me too much until I recalled an experience I had in my mid-twenties, when I was living in Green Valley, Arizona.

I was sitting on the couch beside the front window, which overlooked miles of desert with mountains on the horizon, practicing my daily spiritual exercises.

Suddenly, a spiritual master materialized in my living room. To my surprise I could clearly see the floor-length maroon robe he wore and the back of his bald head.

Instead of turning to look at me, to say hello and share words of great wisdom—which I fully expected he should do—he continued to face away from me.

Why would he do that?

What wrong had I committed that a spiritual master would visit me and keep his back turned?

I felt I was being punished and wore the weight of some unknown guilt like a lead yoke, the full brunt of the unworthiness instilled from my Catholic upbringing. For days, I felt paralyzed by despair.

Finally I reached out for help from a woman who was trained to give spiritual aid. Her name was Millie, and at that time she was living in nearby Tucson. When I phoned her, I explained the visitation I'd had and the nature of my problem. She invited me to her home, where we shared tea.

She then asked me to revisit what happened, moment by moment. I closed my eyes and relived the experience giving her every detail. With the strength of Millie's presence, I staved off the shroud of unworthiness and persisted in the experience.

This time, I noticed things I had not seen before. My knee-jerk guilt reaction had blinded me to the fact that there had been other masters in the room, too. Over a dozen of them! All of them also had their backs to me.

The memory became equally as real as the actual visitation weeks before. Inwardly, I walked up to the masters, said hello and tried to get their attention. Still they ignored me. Again I resisted the temptation of guilt. Ultimately, I turned to look in the direction they were looking.

I cannot recount in words what I then witnessed. The wall of my living room that the masters were facing had become a wall of light, spilling downward like a shimmering waterfall of silvery white. These masters had come to visit me—so that we could together behold the Light of God.

I felt terribly humbled.

As I gazed into the waterfall of light, with my beloved masters at my side, my unworthiness started washing away. It was time to replace it with gratitude. I knew then for certain that I was a child of God, a spark of the divine, a drop in the Ocean of Love and Mercy. I exist because God loves me, and therefore I will accept gratefully all the gifts that God sees fit to bestow upon me—even the ones that are difficult to accept.

By remembering this experience, my belief in my own self-worth evolved from something scented with vanity to something far more humble. I did not feel entitled to a new heart or that I deserved it. Rather, if I lived long enough to receive one, I would accept it with all the gratitude that every cell in my body could possibly muster.

Every day from then on I practiced nurturing gratitude. I wanted to wrap myself in the feeling of being grateful. I wanted to wallow in it.

I believe this feeling of thankfulness may have allowed me to have an emotional-body healing.

One evening, I dreamed I was fully awake and being lifted from my hospital bed. As I rose upward, a sticky wet mud dripped off me. It felt as though I was shedding layers of dross and leaving them forever behind.

A cadre of light-beings surrounded me. They placed my body—I guessed it was my emotional body—onto a stretcher. They didn't carry me; rather, I floated between them.

Since I was lying down, I could not see where we were going. Looking upward, I saw the blue sky, dotted with clouds, and then the tall arched ceiling of an entranceway. The top of a very tall doorway gave way to another enormous ceiling. The ceiling was made of golden bricks and was supported by tall columns, also made of gold.

We moved through this cavernous space and entered a small room with a flat, nondescript white ceiling, probably no more than twice my height. Those who escorted me here looked down at me, encircling me with their beautiful faces, intelligent, and bright. Some were old, some young, and all were peaceful and smiling. Somehow I knew that they were doctors and they were about to perform a procedure.

Would they give me anesthesia here? I doubted it, so I lulled myself into a deeper repose. While I was intensely curious what they were going to do, another part of me preferred not to witness it too closely. I rested my attention on the whiteness of the ceiling and let my mind go blank.

By the sensations I felt in my chest, I guessed they were doing something to release my emotional-body heart and replace it with a new one. This emotional-body heart transplant operation was not without feelings of intensity that one might associate with pain, although physically I felt none. I resisted the temptation to squirm and held my physical body as still as possible.

In time, I felt new life flowing through me.

I awoke in my hospital room, knowing that I had received a special healing. I now felt as tired as I'd ever been, but gone was the anger, hatred, and jealousy, and so many other petty negative emotions that once dogged me so relentlessly. These emotions were somehow tied to my old emotional-body heart. Where did the new one come from? Every answer starts with a question.

Remember when I told you about the time track, and how the causal body separates past, present, and future? As physical doctors can manipulate physical tissue, slice it apart, rearrange it, and sew it back together, my inner-world doctors had similar skills with non-physical fabric. They were able to extract a heart for me from a future incarnation of my own.

They chose an incarnation far enough into the future that represented a lifetime when I had mastered most of the worst negative emotions and no longer chose to experience them. Hence the emotional-body heart they gave me preferred not to express these feelings. The doctors had chosen the moment when my body in that future lifetime died naturally, then they harvested the heart and moved it back on the time track to the moment of now. Then they placed it inside my body—rather, my emotional body.

I had been cleansed and healed, and tremendously blessed. I had just received a new emotional-body heart because my old one was very sick too. No wonder I couldn't even move around in my dream state except in a wheelchair. The cardiac illness I was experiencing was not confined to my physical body. It surpassed it.

How deeply did it go?

The next morning, February 1, 2005, I had an inner conversation with Rebazar about the emotional-body heart transplant I'd received the night before. I hoped it meant I would get a physical heart soon, too.

"You're not ready to receive a new heart," he said matter-of-factly.

I didn't want to hear that. I certainly did not want to believe him.

"I'll be ready," I promised.

I thought of my brother, Paul, who once flew the huge C-5 transport planes in the Air Force. He told me that he never knew when he would be flying. Sometimes they would call him up and he would wait for hours, and then his assignment would be canceled. I reflected on his easy attitude about living with this uncertainty and wondered if I could be as flexible and detached.

When one receives the announcement about a possible donor, it does not guarantee a heart transplant is going to happen. Too many things can get in the way. I could be called to the operating room, prepped for surgery, given anesthesia for it, and wake up learning that something had gone wrong.

To prepare myself, I considered how I would handle the news when they told me of a possible donor. I planned and practiced my response. I would not get excited or too hopeful—so that I wouldn't drown in disappointment if something went wrong. I promised myself I would stay calm and peaceful. I would thank the doctor, who gave me the news. Then, I would think of my spiritual guides and thank them, and God, and the Holy Spirit. Finally, I would surrender to the experience no matter what.

An inner vision later that day helped me take yet another step to readiness. In this lucid dream I saw a forest of vertical columns. They were translucent and covered with symbols. Each was turning one way or the other at its own speed. Each column represented some aspect of my heart transplant experience: my own readiness, plus the readiness of my donor and the donor's family, my family and supporters, and the surgeons involved, plus the readiness of those I might touch in my new life, plus Bob's readiness, and still more. Somehow I knew that when all the moving columns faced forward, the timing would be perfect.

Hours later, I received a vision. Three of the columns turned in unison and fell into place.

I felt alarmed.

I wasn't ready!

* * *

The morning of February 2, 2005, I woke up with the realization that I could talk to my future heart, even when it was still inside my soon-to-be-donor's body. So I extended my attention through time and space to inwardly contact the spiritual intelligence of the donor.

The spirit of the person who would become my donor did not want to talk. However, the Spirit of the Heart—in other words the heart's intelligence—was interested in connecting with me telepathically. Once I put forth the invitation, I could sense the heart spirit reach out to me, curious who I was.

I got straight to the point. "Something both catastrophic and wonderful is going to happen to you—and to me," I said. "Somehow I know for a fact that you need not worry, because the person you live with won't suffer."

The heart sounded relieved to hear this, because it had indeed been worrying. It could sense something was changing in the life energy surrounding its host. It had been bracing itself for the impending unknown.

"You are going to live. And you'll be given a new home inside of my body."

This was information that the heart needed to process. I gave it time in silence to do so, while keeping my attention unwavering.

"My rite of passage will happen before yours," the Spirit of the Soon-to-be-donor's Heart predicted. "But each of us will have to experience one."

A rite of passage. That was a good way to look at it.

When our conversation ended, I knew this would be the last communication I would have with this heart until—if and when—it was mine. In time, anything can happen. Things could shift and this heart might not come to live with me after all.

I turned my attention to my own, native heart. It had a few things it wanted to communicate, too.

"I know I'm limiting our body," my native heart said. "I know I'm sick and making our body sick too. I know I'm going to die."

A sense of peace emanated from it, as though it were an elderly person comfortable with death—just awaiting the right time for its own great transition.

"I am ready to leave."

I said, "I hope that, when you're removed from my body, that you'll be able to teach doctors something that will save other people's lives." A well of emotion emerged, moistening my eyes. "That would be my wish."

"It would be mine, too," my heart replied.

On behalf of my heart, I then sent a prayer into the universe: "As the surgeon lifts you out of my body, may the Angel of Organs lift you into her hands and carry you to heaven."

I am convinced there is a heaven for the organ spirits. Didn't I see an angel carry away the Spirit of my Gallbladder? If organs are intelligent beings as we are, and if we have a heaven, why not them too? I cannot imagine what it might look like, yet I know it exists. I wanted my heart to find a home there, and a new way to serve life, one that it would enjoy after being such a good partner with me all these years.

Thank you heart!

That night, as I fell asleep, I finally felt ready to let go of my dear old heart. For the first time since I had been in the hospital, I was ready to ask for a new heart.

Inwardly, bravely, boldly, I visualized the Healing Council sitting around their long oak table. I approached them and stood at the table's foot.

I recalled a way to ask for miracles that I'd heard an inspirational speaker share from the stage. I decided to use Anne Archer Butcher's technique. I said, "May I please have a heart tomorrow, and if not, then something better?"

The next morning, I was awakened bright and early by a young doctoral fellow new to my team. He walked into my room eager to share an announcement. His tone of voice was upbeat and positive.

"I have really good news."

A heart?

It was 5:30 a.m. While I was still groggy from not sleeping well the night before, I felt instantly hopeful and was immediately alert.

"Your team has decided to replace your I.V. lidocaine with oral procainamide. That means that you'll be going home! You won't need to wait here in the hospital for a heart."

Was I having a nightmare?

He continued, "A few hours ago we started lowering the

dose of lidocaine going into your veins. You'll start taking the oral meds with breakfast."

I could not believe my ears.

"Are they crazy?" I said. I sat up as swiftly as my body would let me.

He looked taken aback. Clearly he did not expect my reaction.

"We tried this at the other hospital. Twice," I explained. "Each time it led to a v-tach storm, and once, a near-death experience."

He looked at me quizzically and said not another word while he checked my vital signs.

Later that morning, I spoke with my cardiologist. She said that my team had decided this course of action was best for me.

"Aren't I supposed to be part of my own team?" I begged her to return the intravenous dose to its previous amount. My pleas did not change her mind.

This was such a lonely journey. Despite my wondrous inner experiences, I still had a lot to learn. Was I being tested? If so, I was not handling it well. I wept uncontrollably and braced myself for an impending v-tach.

My doctors were curious: Why did the news make me so emotional?

More than once, I explained what had happened previously. The lidocaine was my life preserver. I relied on it. Without it, I was doomed. Apparently, all my records were left at the previous hospital because when I asked my doctors to review what had happened the last time my lidocaine was lowered, they looked at me with blank stares.

I resolved to prepare myself for a v-tach storm. Mentally, this was harder than preparing for heart transplant surgery. Emotionally, it was nearly impossible. I fell into depression. My emotional body became like a big blank pit and swallowed me. I moved back and forth between feeling numb and then crying because the emotions were so overwhelming.

The transplant coordinator popped her head in and said she'd like to come by tomorrow to go over transplant details. I said, "Sure, anytime." But I was thinking, "Why bother? What's the point? If they send me home, I'm not going to make it to transplant."

Later that day, the truth surfaced. My transplant nurse told me that my insurance company was badgering the hospital administrators. They insisted it was taking too long to get me a new heart. I began to feel angry toward the insurance company employees who were pressuring my doctors to release me from the hospital. I wanted to ask them where they thought hearts came from? Perhaps someone from the insurance company might want to donate one themselves?

I felt angry toward the doctors, too. Why couldn't they take the time to read my records from the previous hospital and get it through their highly-educated heads that taking me off lidocaine does not work?

I told them they were giving me a death sentence.

They responded by sending in a psychiatrist.

The hospital psychiatrist pestered me about being afraid of death. I kept trying to explain that it wasn't death that frightened me. Been there, done that. What had me so upset was my distaste for the prolonged agony of repeated I.C.D. shocks due to uncontrollable and unpredictable v-tach. I do not know why she didn't seem to understand this. Or she just wasn't listening. She simply asked once again, "Are you afraid to die?"

If they were going to send me home, I seriously considered asking them to turn off the I.C.D. I'd much rather feel over-caffeinated for a while and then slip into the gray zone and have a peaceful death than the torture of unrelenting I.C.D. shocks.

To let go of my angry feelings, I took a few extra laps around the pod. I went around twelve times for a total of half a mile. Feeling calm again, I returned to my room, laid on my bed and my heart promptly fell into v-tach. My faithful heart monitor recorded it for all to see.

The nurses rushed into my room, "How are you feeling?"

"I don't care."

The nurses began to work on me.

This time, I wasn't going to fight the arrhythmia. I'd just let it happen. If my heart wanted us both to die right then, I was totally fine with that. Instead, I got an extra dose of lidocaine in my I.V. and after two minutes, the v-tach was over. Fortunately it passed without the I.C.D. firing.

Am I doomed or blessed to find something to be grateful for in every situation? In this one, I knew that if I had reacted to the v-tach with fear, a flood of hormones could have made the "event" a real party, complete with the lightning-bolt-like fireworks of I.C.D. shocks. Another point of gratitude I could squeeze from this rock resulted in a bit of humor. The longer I hung around until transplant, the more interesting my story would be...if I lived to write it. I tried to laugh at my own joke.

Later that day, another doctor on my team announced that they would reinstate my previous dose of intravenous lidocaine because they didn't know what they were going to do with me. My team would have a meeting to discuss it sometime in the next few days.

Somehow, the experience also left me with a sense of detachment. My daughter, AriaRay, has a term for crying. She calls it "leaking salty water." The next day, February 3, when my primary cardiologist came to visit, I watched myself leak a lot of salty water. I told her that if they wanted me to be part of the team that managed my care (their promise from the beginning), then they needed to let me know about the decisions they wanted to make about me—before they made them. At least they could run an idea by me first, and let me think about it and air my concerns before a decision was made.

She apologized about lowering the lidocaine without talking to me about it first. Then she emphasized that we did need to develop a good relationship, because, she assured me, I was indeed a part of the team. Not just before transplant—but afterward too. The transplant journey would be lifelong. Not only would I be visiting my team regularly for the rest of my life, I would be taking immune-suppressant medicines too. These drugs would subdue my immune system so that it did not try to attack my heart and cause rejection.

I was curious about the side effects of these drugs.

"Ninety-nine percent of the people who take them get side effects, for which nothing can be done," she said. "These side effects include: shaking hands, extra hair growth, loss of appetite, and stomach trouble. Other side effects get treated as soon as they come up, such as high cholesterol, high blood pressure, diabetes, and cancer." She explained that cancer was the primary cause of death for heart transplant patients because of the immune system suppression.

I was still leaking salty water when our conversation ended.

My doctor reminded me to sing HU, and sang it for me while I sobbed.

19

WE TRADE HEARTS

My transplant team had done its best to make me as comfortable as possible during the time while I waited for my new heart. One of the nicest things the team did was to reduce the number of times they requested a blood draw from twice a day to once a day, to finally, every other day. This was a blessing because I was seriously running out of real estate on my hands and arms from which the blood could be taken.

Both my right and left forearms and hands had become so bruised and swollen that I needed to sleep with a special heating pad wrapped around them. Eventually, the veins in my hands and arms got so bad they were unusable for drawing blood. So the doctors inserted a pic line into a vein near my right clavicle, where they could tap my blood at any time.

The other really nice thing they did was to fulfill my request for a sign on my door that read:

"DO NOT DISTURB Between 10:00 p.m. and 6:00 a.m."

If they wanted me strong enough for transplant, I told them, I needed sleep. Without this sign to stop them, people would barge into my room at all hours of the night, turn on the bright overhead lights without warning, and then prick, probe, weigh, measure, interrogate, and check, giving me precious little time to rest. With eight hours all to myself, I found some peace. Because I value my privacy and had consecrated my hospital room as sacred space, this time meant more to me than you could possibly imagine.

On Friday, February 4, 2005, I was looking forward to seeing Bob again. He had finally overcome the flu. Usually, he would spend the night at a hotel. Since I hadn't seen him for so long, I convinced him to sleep on a cot in my hospital room.

Bob had been by my side since my heart first failed in October, 2002. He had persevered through all my medical trials and put his entire life aside to be there for me in every way. It was no coincidence he was with me again on this night.

He brought some special food with him. We enjoyed various hors d'oeuvres and goodies. I relished anything besides hospital food. We went to bed about 10:30 p.m. and I finally fell asleep about 1:00 a.m.

An hour later, two doctors walked in, abruptly turned on the overhead lights, and stood at the foot of my bed.

My first thought (and I may have said it aloud, too), was an indignant, "Didn't you see the sign on the door?"

"We're surgeons from the transplant team, and we think we've found a heart for you."

"Wow."

That was my very first reaction.

Then I dutifully said the gratitude prayer I'd been practicing for this very moment. I could hardly believe I actually had the opportunity to say it for real.

The problem was, I couldn't quite say the prayer exactly as I planned it. The word "wow" kept creeping in every few words. I felt awash in a miracle, and it was overwhelming.

"We have you scheduled for surgery in six hours," the surgeons said. They explained that I'd be called for an x-ray in a couple of hours. I would have some other prep work to do, and then an hour before surgery they would take me to pre-op.

Bob asked where the heart was coming from and how it was going to get here.

They said the heart was coming from an automobile accident victim in another state. A surgical team from my hospital was flying down to harvest the heart. They had to work with other teams who would be harvesting other donated organs first, such as kidneys and liver. The heart is needed to keep these other organs alive, they explained, and so it would come out last.

If the heart looked good, they would telephone the team back here. Both my surgical teams—the one here and the one there—would confirm that everything was still a "go." If so, they would pack the heart in ice and place it in an ordinary lunch cooler. Then, time was of the essence, as they would have only four hours to get the heart back inside a body—my body.

The team that had gone to the donor's hospital would come home by the fastest means possible. They would take an ambulance or helicopter to the nearest airport where a chartered jet would await them. Airspace would be cleared for a direct flight to my local airport, where a helicopter would meet them to race the heart back to my hospital.

By the time the heart arrived, my chest cavity would be open and I would be fully prepared to release my dear, old, worn-out heart and receive the new, healthy heart.

"Try to get some sleep," the surgeons said and left.

Sleep? That was impossible. I was so excited.

I worked very hard to keep calm. The last thing I needed was for another episode of arrhythmia that might kill me before my new heart was implanted. Although I was sure that, if my heart failed at this point, they would find a way to keep me going until the operation.

The meeting with the surgeons had been surreal. I laughed aloud. Of all days for this to happen, it was the day that Bob was finally here. It was the first night he had ever slept in my room in this hospital and also the weekend the spiritual teaching I followed was holding a seminar in a nearby town.

I felt Spirit was with me.

Before I was called down for the pre-op preparations, I was able to doze. While I slept, I had an inner-world experience with my donor.

I found myself in the Peaceful Place. Nothing in particular caught my attention. I was just content to be there. Then, from out of the gray mist I saw a woman running toward me wearing a hospital gown. Her arms were stretched wide as though she wanted to hug me. Her face was bright, and she was smiling widely.

We recognized each other instantly, although I do not remember ever seeing her before. As she drew nearer, I opened my arms to embrace her. Just as I felt the warmth of her body against mine, she passed through me as though we were both ghosts.

I turned around to look where she had gone. She stood a few yards away, still facing me and still smiling. In her outstretched hands she held my poor, enlarged, and very sick heart. As she passed through me, she had swapped it for her own.

"Take my heart with you to heaven?" I asked. "Perhaps, to a special heaven just for organs?"

She nodded in agreement. Then she waved, turned, and continued her journey into the Light.

When I wrote this experience to the donor family, my mother suggested I not use any pronouns out of respect for the family—because what if the donor was male? Here, I wanted to relay the experience as I remembered it. If I ever discover my donor was male, then I'll have to admit that I do not know why I saw my donor as a woman.

* * *

When we arrived in pre-op before dawn on Saturday morning, February 5, 2005, the usually bustling room was empty. I met my surgeon, who was the same doctor who had repaired my heart's valves the previous year. He was bright-eyed and alert, and paced the floor energetically, sporting the biggest cup of Starbucks I'd ever seen.

I realized the reason for his electric enthusiasm. He was about to perform heart-transplant surgery—not something that's done every day. The hospital averaged only one or two per month. My surgeon's positive attitude boosted my confidence.

Waiting in pre-op, I was not nervous, worried, or anxious. I was just exceedingly joyful. It was one of the happiest days of my life. I felt so very blessed and grateful—even though I knew something could go against the plan. I might wake up without the new heart or I might wake up in heaven. It was win-win either way.

Finally it was time to go to the operating room. I said goodbye to Bob and refocused on my coming adventure. Despite my near-death experience, I still felt I needed courage. I repeated a line over and over again from a favorite book, *Stranger by the River*, by Paul Twitchell. I'd memorized it for the occasion:

Fill thyself with Light, and death cannot overtake thee.

No matter what happened, it was important to me that my attention remain on the Light. If I was going to transition for good this time, I wanted to be fully aware of my journey. Death would not obliterate me if my attention remained on the Light, because I'd retain my awareness through the transition.

As I continued to repeat the sentence I'd memorized, it shifted to this, "I fill myself with Light, and death cannot overtake me." By the time I was moved to the operating table, my mantra was this, "I am the Light and death cannot overtake me."

The anesthesiologists began to prep me for their part of the operation. I knew I'd be unconscious soon. I asked the chief anesthesiologist, who sat behind my head, if he would do me a favor.

"Sure," he said. "If I can."

"When the entire surgical team is here, would you tell them 'thank you' for me?"

"That's not a request I get very often."

"Please don't forget to tell them."

In the unconscious state of general anesthesia, time passes without you realizing it. Yet some of the memories of what happened in between falling asleep and waking up remain.

I remember someone making an inappropriate comment about my anatomy during the pre-op prep. My anesthesiologist reprimanded him; in my view, not severely enough.

I remember the bustle in the room when the surgeons showed up with the heart. At this time, I moved from my post hovering behind my anesthesiologist's shoulder to a new one behind my surgeon's. It was odd to hear my sternum being sawed apart, and to see my chest wide open, with the organs inside. I remember thinking, "Is that really me under there?" I was covered head to toe with surgical cloths.

When the new heart was sewn in place, I watched as everyone waited with baited breath for the heart to start pumping. This suspended moment offered me one last choice-point: did I really want to go back? The spiritual masters standing on both sides of me would accommodate any choice I made—although they explained there would be karmic repercussions with the donor if I chose not to accept the gift.

I only half heard them, as my attention was transfixed on the heart now inside my chest. It looked so beautiful. I wanted to get to know it better.

"Why waste a good heart?" I said telepathically.

Just then my new heart started beating. Those in attendance whooped and cheered and got to work closing my ribcage.

*   *   *

I awoke in the recovery room late that afternoon, although I had zero sense of what time it was. Bob was there with my dad. We had called my parents as soon as we had been informed about the potential donor. My father had taken the first flight out of Houston Saturday morning. I was surprised and glad that he had arrived so quickly. It was comforting to have my small but faithful support team with me.

My foremost concern was a tremendous longing to communicate something. The breathing tube down my throat prevented this, and the nurse kept saying I was nauseous. I wasn't nauseous. I just wanted to talk except that my efforts sounded like I was gagging. My inability to speak bothered me even more than the fact that my arms were strapped beside me.

Luckily Bob knew immediately what I wanted and got out a pen and paper. They untied my arms and he held the pad as I tried to write. He has kept the notes I made. They are endearing, humorous, and mostly illegible insights into the perceptions of a loopy, still-half-anesthetized mind.

Unfortunately, most of what I wrote had to do with trying to convince the nurse I wasn't nauseous and would they please remove the breathing tube? The urgent message that I was trying so hard to communicate was lost. I hope to remember it someday, as I believe it was a message from my donor.

20

POST-TRANSPLANT CHALLENGES

"*I* can't breathe!" I screamed silently when they removed the breathing tube. My chest felt impossibly heavy, as though loaded with bricks. I searched the room for the nurse.

"You can do it," she said.

I looked into her eyes, "No, I can't," I thought. My lungs had forgotten how to work. A wave of terror passed through me and I feared suffocation. I gasped, inefficiently. Little by little, I had to learn all over again how to coordinate my muscles to inhale properly. Once I did, I fell back to sleep.

One of my next memories was the feeling of something warm flooding my veins. I opened my eyes and saw a nurse adjusting a bag of dark red fluid on an I.V. stand.

"Is that blood?"

"You lost a lot during the operation. I'm giving you two pints."

I was awake enough to think and my thoughts ran wild. Where did the blood come from? What had its donor's diet been like??

When I felt my life-energy rise like the gas gauge that moves up when you fill your car's gas tank, I brushed aside my concerns. The blood was too revitalizing and deeply life-giving for any of them to matter. I opened my heart completely to receive this new blood and sent gratitude into the universe to whomever the donor had been. Never had I felt so physically nourished at such a deep and fundamental level.

The next day they moved me out of the I.C.U. and into a private room. Among my first visitors were the physical therapists.

"You're going to climb some stairs today."

"You're kidding me."

I tried to plea my case: I'd just come out of major heart surgery and was flanked by two I.V. poles, one at each side of my head, each stacked with bags of medicines. I felt fully entrenched between them.

"We're not kidding."

I thought their tone sounded a little mischievous.

They deftly switched the I.V. poles to portable ones, while I heaved myself out of bed. This wasn't easy because I had four, half-inch-wide chest tubes protruding out of my abdomen. They had been inserted into my lungs during the surgery to drain excess fluid and were temporarily sealed with two foot-long, very heavy, scissor-like clamps. The tubes snaked through a vacuum pump into a large fluid collection container. To go for a walk, I had to carry both the clamps and my heart monitor, while my physical therapists waddled along beside me carrying the vacuum pump and canister, and pushing the two loaded I.V. poles.

What a circus.

At first, I shuffled into the hallway. When I realized that walking was easy and pain-free, I straightened my posture. We walked around the pod.

"Time to climb some steps."

"I can't."

"You can."

I rolled my eyes. I hadn't been able to walk up a step in months. What were they thinking? I intended to humor them—and prove them wrong.

I put a foot on one step and lifted myself onto the next. Then another, and then another.

"I can!" I exclaimed, completely astonished. "I'm not even out of breath!" I wanted to walk up more, and the physical therapists allowed me another three.

I was elated. This was fantastic! Unbelievable! Two days ago, I couldn't even think of climbing a step. No longer did I care how many drugs were dripping into my veins. I was going to get my life back. I would see my children again.

A day or two later, I was weaned down one I.V. pole. A few days after that, all the I.V.s were removed and I was switched to oral medications. For breakfast, they handed me two one-ounce medicine cups—I kid you not—filled to the brim with pills. They consisted of immune-suppressants, antibiotics, anti-virals, antifungals, medicines for my heart, vitamins and minerals, and medicines to protect my stomach from all the other medicines.

How on earth was I going to deal with this?

When I was a teenager and young adult, my friends were into natural living. Many of them vocally denounced the medical profession. They deplored allopathic drugs, which when they killed people, resulted in no more than a slap on the wrist of the pharmaceutical companies that had made them. Whereas, if such a thing happened to an herbal company, they'd be out of business and their owners thrown in jail. Through these discussions, I always held my tongue. I knew the medical profession had its place—just as much as the alternative methods did. Maybe a part of me knew my life would one day depend on the allopaths and their drugs. I found myself thanking myself for never having held a bad attitude about this profession. That being said, I still had two large piles of pills to swallow.

I stared at the medicines and they seemed to stare back. Then I noticed that I could find a pill representing each color of the rainbow in these two little cups. No longer were they potential poisons; they were containers of life-giving colors that would help me stay alive and thrive.

Fortunately I knew how to swallow several pills at once. Otherwise, it would have taken me the entire day to get them down—just in time for the evening doses.

The meds were the price of life. It was my duty and responsibility to take them. I also felt it was an obligation to my donor family. Inwardly, I promised them that I would keep this body as healthy as I possibly could. It was the new home of their loved one's heart. This was the best way I knew to honor their gift.

I know how powerful beliefs are and decided that beyond fulfilling the purpose these meds were meant to serve, they would not affect my body in any negative way. I truly believed this and still do.

Before transplant, one of the doctors on my transplant team was concerned about how my spiritual path might interfere with my taking the meds. The literature he had read about it emphasized the importance of an individual's trust and reliance on inner guidance.

One day he confronted me, "What if your spiritual guide tells you to stop taking the meds? Will you listen?"

I told him what he wanted to hear, though I was offended by the question. How was my path any different from any other when it came to listening inwardly to one's spiritual guide? Did he ask his Christian patients if they would stop taking their meds if Jesus asked them to stop?

Fortunately, my chief cardiologist, who had an Indian heritage, found similarities between the teaching I followed and her own Eastern one. She assuaged the other doctor's concerns and defended my beliefs. I doubted very much that my spiritual guidance would ever tell me to stop taking the meds, and to this day, it never has.

Nevertheless, the effects of the post-transplant drugs were not easy to deal with and played havoc with my motor control. The doctors and nurses, while helpful in other ways, ignored questions they could not answer, such as how long would it be before my legs would stop shaking? Or, will I ever be able to hold a pen and write legibly again?

The few notes I did manage to scrawl in my journal—those which I am able to decipher—talk about the first week following transplant being a "dark night of Soul." I'm certain this was an effect of the high doses of drugs they had started me off with. A heart transplant patient I'd spoken with at the previous hospital had assured me, "If you can get through the first six months, you'll be fine." It's during this time that the doctors gradually reduce the meds or your body simply gets accustomed to them.

Meanwhile, my usually cheerful and positive outlook eluded me, and I felt mired in a funk. Each time I was able to pull out of it, I could see the perfect timing involved and the grace in the experience. These moments were rare, and I often acted in ways that didn't seem like me.

When the surgeon who performed the transplant visited, I wanted to thank him for his part in this wonderful gift. Instead, all I could do was to complain about the fact that my limbs would not stop shaking, and why weren't they removing the awful chest tubes?

As my mind and body cleared from the anesthesia, the pain and discomfort of the chest tubes became more obvious. The surgical team regularly x-rayed my chest to see how well my lungs were healing. If they saw progress, they would let the tubes "water drain" for several hours, clamp them for several more hours, and then take another x-ray.

If the team was not satisfied with the healing progress, the clamps would come off and the vacuum pump would go on. My next twelve hours would be hell. I'd drown in pain and be unable to move or eat.

Throughout my hospital stay, my blood results consistently showed I was nutritionally depleted. Partly this was because, due to my weakened heart, I'd had no appetite. Now that I had a new heart, my dietician insisted that I eat more to regain strength. While I was now much more interested in food, I found the salt-free, fat-free cardiac diet unappetizing.

"I'll make a deal with you," I told my dietician. "If you let me have some butter and sour cream on my baked potato, I promise to eat the whole thing plus the steak that comes with it."

Finally she relented. It was a hard-won arrangement because of her concern about the salt and fat. Needless to say, the entire day, I looked forward to butter and sour cream. My mouth watered when the meal arrived. My stomach might have growled too with anticipation.

Just as I was about to take my first bite, the results of the latest x-ray also came in. A nurse turned on the vacuum pump.

"Can't you wait until I finish eating?"

"Nope."

Where was the teamwork that was supposed to be happening among my benefactors?

The coveted meal sat uneaten beside my bed while I sank into agony, hungry. I felt doubly awful that my dietician would notice the uneaten meal. She recorded everything I ate. I had let her down and broken an agreement. She never visited me again.

That night, the pain from the chest tubes seemed especially unbearable.

I pleaded for painkillers.

"Your organs have yet to recover from the anesthesia you had during surgery" the doctors said. "Giving you painkillers will only make that process more difficult."

At about 4:00 a.m., I was suffering so much that I called Dad at his hotel room to appeal on my behalf for pain management. He came over right away. His efforts were unsuccessful. The doctors simply would not give me analgesics. My dad stayed with me that entire day until late that night. He sat in my room reading and being a comforting presence. Loving me without words.

Telling you how grateful I was for my dad's presence doesn't scratch the surface of how deeply touched I felt about this quiet gesture.

Looking back on these circumstances, I remember complaining about the pain, and then simply dealing with it. I didn't get upset, angry, or frustrated. I met the situation, sank into the pain, and coped. I relied heavily on thinking HU. I didn't have the strength to sing it.

A breakthrough occurred when one of the doctoral fellows described to me exactly why the chest tubes were there. He explained my lungs had not yet healed from my previous surgery a year ago. The tissue was still torn. Unless these tears were sealed, I could drown in my own fluids without the tubes to drain them.

So I began an unrelenting effort to constantly imagine that the lung tissue where the tears were located had turned to butter, and that a golden butter knife was gently smoothing the cells back into place. I am sure this sped up my healing process.

The next day, the surgeons took out the two tubes on the left, and soon after they removed the two that remained on the right. The tubes came out fast, and the breathing pattern I was given to do during their removal was sufficiently distracting. It didn't hurt, and I would have rated it only "moderate" on the queasy scale until I saw the length of the tubes that had been inside me. They were about three feet long!

I did not expect to feel so free without them. Finally I could reclaim the boundaries of my own body, and immediately I started to feel better and gain strength.

On the twelfth day post-transplant, my surgeon said that from the surgical team's viewpoint I was ready to go home. I just needed permission from the transplant team.

What joy!

As soon as he left my room, I phoned the transplant nurse with the news.

She said "Why not tomorrow? Can Bob be here by noon?"

After eighty-one days in the hospital, I would be going home!

Over the past weeks and months, I had developed many routines that had helped me cope and keep a positive attitude. On this final day in the hospital, I revisited every one, knowing it would be my last. Every little experience or visit by a doctor, nurse, patient-care assistant or phlebotomist, I was counting down as the last, and blessing it as the last, and thanking God it would be the last.

Throughout this past week, Rebazar remained at my side and members of the Healing Council had visited me often to check in and see how I was doing. Sadly, I was unable to visit the Great Library. I needed to hold vigil over myself—to be my own Guardian Angel.

On my final night before leaving the hospital, I was about to fall asleep, when one of the members of the Healing Council, dressed in white, approached me with an announcement. I usually perceived these beings floating on the ceiling. This time, he stepped down into my reality and stood near the foot of my bed.

Later, I would learn he was the Guardian of White Sapphire. He was a big man, both in size and height, with tan skin and thick wavy white hair falling just to his shoulders. His big, bright brown eyes showed well-disciplined strength and determination.

"You will no longer be transcribing in the Great Library," he said in a deep, resonant voice. "Soon, your work will continue on the physical plane. However, you are welcome to return to the library at any time to review what you have recorded, as well as the research others have done."

"I don't want to give up my job."

"There is healing to be done and responsibility to take."

I assumed he was talking about my healing journey. Yet his message seemed broader than that. He was talking about the personal and the universal at once.

"People today have needs unknown to those of previous generations," he said. "They are faced with challenges brought about by their environment and by their own kind. The Earth is changing on its own, and by hands of human intervention. Food, air, and water are being compromised as never before.

"At the same time, people are ready to return to a new Golden Age. They are ready to learn how to take care of themselves: to master the life-giving energy flows that move through them, to nourish themselves with color rays, and to protect themselves from all that would steal life energies away."

"Is this what I'm supposed to do?" I wasn't sure what he was saying or why.

"Those who are most purely and uniquely themselves have the most to offer this world. They are the leaders, the light bearers, the inventors, and successful creatives of society. Do I speak of people? Yes, but this is true of other life forms as well. The herbs whose energies are most unique and definitive have the greatest healing benefits. The cells most true to their functions enjoy the greatest health. Superlatives come with uniqueness and self-assuredness.

"Any pure energy form will be powerful and promote change. The changes can be positive if you apply the energies for purposes of healing. They can be destructive if you use them for self-empowerment or to change others against their will."

He paused, as though giving me some time for the words to sink in, and then continued.

"The Earth's crystals have exceedingly pure energies and have been used both positively and negatively in the past. Some of the negative ways have led to massive destruction. That's why you and many others feel uncomfortable or wary of them today. You have experienced this misuse in the past, in previous incarnations.

"We of the Healing Council keep safely stored the records of the ways and methods by which crystals were used destructively. You and others of your world may now have access to information about their healing properties.

"You know the principle: despise someone of another race, country, or religion, and you will reincarnate yourself into that person's circumstances. Likewise, those who vehemently deny a thing, fear, hate, or distrust it must come back to use it and find peace with it, to neutralize the energies they put forth against it.

"So we have a population ready to experience the healing side of gemstones. Once they took part in destruction, now they must build and correct. The karma belongs not only to the individuals involved, but also to the Earth and her crystals."

I wondered if he was referring to the part crystals played in the destruction of Atlantis.

"Yes," he replied, "even the gemstones have a debt to repay. To serve as healing vehicles provides them the opportunity to correct the wrongs they were once involved in—even against their will."

When the Guardian finished, he touched my forehead briefly and gently, and then moved back toward the ceiling and through the heavenly window that appeared there.

I was left alone to ponder one question: Why did he tell me this?

Years later, I realized that my heart transplant was a key part of my gemstone journey. It was essential for me to fulfill my mission in this lifetime. For whatever reason, the heart I was born with was attached to karma of the unworthy. Even when I believed unworthiness was not my issue, it was.

It's one thing to feel as though you don't deserve something. It's another to have something at your fingertips and not step up to the responsibility. In the late 1980s, I had been given the perfect opportunity to bring Diamond and Gemstone Therapy to the planet. For whatever reason, I wasn't ready to take charge of my own mission and purpose. I like to think the world wasn't ready—except that only takes the blame off my own shoulders.

Yes, perhaps it's a better story this way. Certainly I appreciate life far more than I ever could have without a heart transplant. Maybe it all worked out the way it was supposed to.

What I do know is that I stepped out of the hospital a new person. I had shed so much emotional and mental baggage, and found a resource of inner strength and determination I didn't know I had. Perhaps it took something as dramatic as a heart transplant for me to step closer to my full potential.

Inner transformations can take time to manifest. Foremost, I had a lot of healing yet to do. I also needed to remember my gemstone mission and accept my destiny.

21

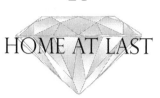

HOME AT LAST

*B*ob has a special way of making a house feel like a home. When I walked through the door for the first time with my new heart, everything looked clean and tidy. I took a moment to breathe in the familiar scent. Every home has its own. Our small Cape Cod-style home was flavored with wood floors, wallpaper, and oriental carpets.

I walked through one room and then the next, moving carefully, as though holding myself together. It would take many weeks before it felt as though the pieces of my body were back in place, and I felt physically integrated. While I was not in pain, my body felt as stiff as a board.

I found my favorite armchair in the living room and sat down to rest while Bob went to do errands. Plants lined the table in front of our picture window, and I gazed peacefully at the familiar artwork on our walls.

Rest did not come easily. The heating system cranked itself on, and I jumped at the noise—fully expecting someone to walk in—like at the hospital. I realized I needed to shed the anxiety of hospital life and trade it for the peace of living at home. Never again would I be wakened at dawn by a phlebotomist keen on drawing blood or a doctoral fellow on his morning rounds.

"I have something for you," Bob announced when he returned. "Prepare yourself."

I went to the kitchen to find two full grocery bags on the table.

"Food?" I felt ravenous.

"Your meds."

I sat down, feeling dazed. While Bob unpacked the bags, I stared at the growing piles of medicine bottles and boxes on the table. They would need to be sorted and organized into daily doses. The pharmacy also sent over a blood-glucose test kit, which I would have to learn to use.

Now I knew why the transplant nurse thought I'd need a bigger support team. The job felt overwhelming. What might have taken someone else thirty minutes took me three hours—not including a nap in the middle. Bob had to leave for a meeting and couldn't help me. The job forced me to gather my energies and practice mental discipline and focus. In the end, it was a good exercise.

That evening, I felt especially disoriented. Torn from my hospital routines, I did not know what to do with myself and began wandering aimlessly from room to room. I ended up in the bathroom, staring in the mirror at my scars.

An inch-wide red line ran from my collarbone down to my stomach. I was held together with surgical glue, which would eventually wash off in the shower. Under my ribcage, I had four bright red gashes from the chest tubes, and four others from the previous surgery, which had already healed into white lines. Four small red lines on my right abdomen reminded me of my gallbladder removal surgery.

Under my right collarbone, my skin was marred with a three-inch long incision that I was surprised to find when I awoke from the surgery. It was where the life-support apparatus had been inserted.

186

Under my left collarbone, I now had four scars where I.C.D. units had been inserted. When my transplant surgeon told me he would make the fourth incision to remove the last I.C.D., I asked if he would superimpose it onto the scar of the third. This way, the set of three scars would look more like the letter "Z." This letter had a special meaning for me, and I felt comforted to be wearing it.

Many scars on my left and right groin marked insertions into veins during the transplant and the two failed ablation operations and for artery access during angiograms. Of course, my hands and forearms were dotted with small scars from the I.V. insertions, and my neck was riddled with scars where veins were accessed for I.V.s, pic lines, and biopsy catheters.

It looked as though I'd been in a fencing match and lost.

One of our favorite musicians, Steven Wilson, wrote a song with the lyrics: "All I have left are my precious scars." I looked forward to the day when this would be my truth too.

My body was also covered with old adhesive tape from I.V.s, electrocardiogram leads, heart monitor leads, the pic line, and who knows what else. The tape smelled like the hospital, and I couldn't wait to get it off me. I would spend hours rubbing it from my skin. It would take about a week before I was completely free of it.

Bob found me in the bathroom.

I covered myself. "I'm damaged."

Could he, would he, still love me?

"You're not damaged, just decorated," he replied and kissed me.

Then we marveled at my surgeon's fine work.

When we had finished staring at my scars, it was time for bed. Lying down was an exercise in logistics. How does one get horizontal with the least amount of pain? I didn't have the automatic reclining bed that I had in the hospital to help me get there.

Once I got horizontal, it was equally difficult to turn onto one side. Before I did so, I had to ask myself if a new position was really worth the struggle to get there. It would be three weeks before I could roll over in bed pain free—if I was careful enough.

On this first night back home, with my body finally in a comfortable position, I let go one last sigh and closed my eyes.

Suddenly, my vision was filled with light.

I was back beyond the veil of death!

This was quite the surprise. I knew I wasn't dying—the strong, steady beat of my heart assured me of that. What was going on?

The light met me and surrounded me. I felt welcomed in this world of light, and I re-lived the highlights of my near-death experience. Then, I simply reveled in the Light, as one might soak for a long time in a nice hot bath. After about an hour or two, the experience faded, and I slipped into sleep.

Night after night this continued. Every time I closed my eyes to go to sleep, I found myself encompassed by the brightest Light and sweetest Sound. It was comforting, healing, and renewing. I did not ask the Light any questions. I did not want anything from it, nor did I expect it to do anything for me. I simply watched it, and I felt as though It might be watching me, too.

Only when I look back on this experience do I realize it was out of the ordinary. At the time, it felt natural and normal. Nor did I ever guess it might evolve into something that required physical note-taking, or that it would lead me into an entirely new chapter of my life. This, however, would take over a year to unfold.

As the Guardian of White Sapphire had told me, "There was healing to be done and responsibility to take."

I started taking responsibility by spending about an hour

every day talking with my organs. I loved this peaceful, intro-spective time. I began with my heart. I placed my hands over it, welcomed it home, and thanked it for being with me.

"You have experienced some remarkable changes," I said to my heart. "You'll need to recover and take time to grieve the loss of your previous host."

Then I sent it love, and I sensed it was received.

I wanted my heart to feel protected. "Now that you have completed your own rite of passage, you are safe," I reassured it.

Then, with one hand over my heart, I would place my oth-er hand over other parts of my body one at a time. With each placement, I would introduce my heart to my other organs, and vice versa. I would do three or four organs at a time. With each introduction, I would invite us to be together for as long as we lived. This statement seemed very reassuring to all.

Sometimes instead of repeating the introductions, I would simply pass my hand from one part of my body to another, thanking each organ and body part for keeping me alive. If I felt so inspired, I would ask my heart and my other organs how they were doing and if they wanted to say anything.

"Lungs were my first friend," my heart once told me. The news was unexpected and assured me I was not making this up.

"Heart got scared when we were on the heart-lung machine," Lungs said.

"So Lungs comforted me," Heart said. "Lungs had been on that machine before, and assured me that everything would be okay. And it was."

"I'm ignoring Heart," the Spirit of my Immune System an-nounced.

"Is this because of the anti-rejection meds?"

"Yes. Also, I'm aware of my protective role. I know I need to leave our new heart alone."

Still, I asked it to watch out for anything that didn't belong in or around the heart, and it agreed.

To my surprise, the tissues on my right shoulder, where the unexpected incision was made during the transplant were terribly angry.

"Would you like to go into a healing chamber?" I asked the spirit of these tissues.

They agreed reluctantly, because inevitably that meant they would have to face their anger and let go of it.

For me, healing chambers usually appear spherical or in the shape of a Platonic solid dominated by a particular color. This one was a sphere and filled with a pale greenish light. The spirit of the scarred tissues relished the opportunity to tell me how they felt, and so once inside the healing chamber I let them scream and shout and vent their feelings. It took several sessions like this before they stopped being angry and settled into acceptance.

My stomach and small intestines were struggling with all the meds, trying to sort out what to accept and what to reject. Meanwhile, my large intestine was still recovering from the anesthesia. Of all my organs, they had taken the biggest hit.

I also began listening to my heart with a stethoscope. I didn't realize how the beating of a strong, healthy heart resounds throughout the chest. What beautiful rhythm. In the years to follow, and especially whenever my heart felt funny, I would take out the stethoscope and listen. Listening to my heart's regular, uninterrupted beat was more comforting than you might imagine. It assured me that everything was okay.

* * *

In April, Dad arrived for a second two-week visit. He asked about the side effects I was experiencing from all the medications.

I reported neuropathy, my swollen face, and my shaking legs and hands. The skipping heartbeats were hardest to deal with. They were discomforting and unnerving. When the skipping occurred every three or four beats, my chest would tighten, my heart would pound, and my head felt light. This spurred waves of anxiety.

I had begun to feel increasingly anxious whenever I left the house. When my Dad took me to renew my expired driver's license, I fought to stay calm. I told myself there is good anxiety and bad anxiety. The good kind protects us, prepares us for new experiences, and keeps us alert. I tried to convince myself that I was feeling good anxiety and to be grateful for it.

At the Department of Motor Vehicles, a clerk processed my paperwork. "Do you want to be an organ donor?"

I almost burst into tears.

"I am an organ recipient. It's because someone else signed their license that I'm alive." I told her how recently I had received my heart.

"My father is alive today because someone gave him a kidney," she said.

We looked into each other's eyes and shared an unspoken gratitude. We both knew first-hand the gift of organ donation.

I signed the form. A small red heart on the front of my drivers' license now denotes that I am a registered donor. If I could save a life, as someone had saved mine...wow, what a perfect ending that would make.

I should also report a positive side effect: waves of elation. Overwhelming feelings of joy would wash through me daily, causing me to stop what I was doing and remember how wonderful it was to be alive. I was so grateful to have a new heart— and to not be living in the hospital anymore. Even now, not a day goes by that I don't think about and appreciate the gift. I don't ever want to take for granted a single day of life—nor any one special moment in it.

At my first echocardiogram post-transplant, I lay on a treatment table, and the technician sat beside me with her computer nearby. We could both see the images on the monitor.

"Can you show me where my new heart was attached?" I asked.

"Here are the sutures." She pointed to certain lines on my right atrium.

Amazing.

She said, "When I started echocardiography twenty years ago, it looked as though heart recipients had two right atria, or else the right atrium looked significantly larger than it should be. Nowadays, with improved surgical technique, the right atrium is truer to size. Yours looks almost normal."

Many thanks to my wonderful surgeon!

It felt good to see my heart face-to-face, beating so rhythmically and looking so healthy.

By day, I struggled with gaining strength, routine tests for rejection, regular setbacks, and a re-integration of my life back into the real world. At night, I'd re-enter the Light. Every night before bed, the Light continued to meet me, no matter what was going on outwardly. Often it would keep me awake for hours before I finally fell asleep. Though I might have complained of insomnia, I did not share its cause.

Beholding the Light never got boring. I'd bask in the peace and the divine intelligence, soaking it up, and letting it have its way with me. By surrendering to it, I'd allow the Light and Sound to penetrate more and more of me and go increasingly deeper into my fabric. Time was meaningless in the presence of this Light. Sometimes fifteen minutes would pass, sometimes an hour or two.

To describe the Sound I must give you opposites. The Sound was both sweet and striking, deep yet high, melodic yet single-noted, and both nourishing and cleansing. I know these experiences were taking place beyond my mind, because these descriptions don't make logical sense.

Nor did I remember anything in particular happening. It was just me and the Light. Face to face. Back to back. Belly to belly. Heart to heart. In moments of honesty I wondered if I didn't remember anything from these inner experiences because I didn't want to remember. Maybe I was still resisting the knowledge the Light was offering. Maybe I just wasn't ready for it.

23

I REMEMBER MY MISSION

When I was in the hospital, my full attention was necessarily on survival. I was blissfully spared having to look at the inner imbalances that were the underlying causes of the heart failure. In the beginning I had asked for the truth. I wasn't ready to see it then.

When I got home, the circumstances were ideal for exploring the real reasons for the heart failure. I knew I had stuff to deal with, but doing so required digging deeply into some muddy places in order to see what was there and clean them out. What was the hurry? I figured I had plenty of time. Without symptoms to urge me on, I decided to wait to get back to normal and then I would do the required self-healing.

Besides, I had bigger life-issues nagging at me. I still had no idea how or where I was going to find work, and I felt unsettled about not being married.

Always another excuse.

I had lost my compass in life, my purpose and my direction. The real me wanted to come out—whomever she was. I blamed the feeling of being disconnected from myself as another symptom of the anti-rejection meds.

My heart knew the truth and was not going to let me ignore it.

One day, on my way home from a short walk, my heart started pounding. I couldn't catch my breath, I felt light-headed, overheated, and suddenly too exhausted to make it back. Fortunately, this happened in front of Jack and Lorraine's house. My neighbors welcomed me in and called Bob, who came to fetch me. The symptoms were scary because they reminded me of the v-tach. I fell into panic, which made things worse. As a result, I spent the rest of that day and the next in bed, totally exhausted.

I know that if you don't figure out the reason for a health concern and address it thoroughly, it will return. My present heart was incapable of ventricular tachycardia, though it could race.

Was my heart trying to tell me something?

If so, what? If this was a dream, what did it mean? I examined the symbols involved. My heart was beating fast. One explanation was that it was in a hurry. I did not know where we were hurrying toward.

Soon afterward, I started to feel light-headed after exercise and also at night. As the weeks progressed, the lightheadedness became more persistent. It would intensify unpredictably and made me feel as though I would pass out. This feeling was accompanied by an odd sensation in my chest, a tightness or pressure that came and went in an unsteady rhythm. The arrhythmic quality of it made me concerned about my heart. The stethoscope assured me my heart sounded fine—except for a missed beat here and there.

My cardiologist ordered another echocardiogram. It showed a perfectly normal heart. It also revealed some very good news: Whereas before the transplant my ejection fraction had been six (normal is fifty-five) it was now seventy.

I had traded in my clunker for a Ferrari!

I certainly had a powerful engine in me now. Nonetheless, by the end of the week, the chest sensations and lightheadedness were almost constant. It was hard to leave the house because I didn't know if I was going to pass out.

One evening the lightheadedness came on so strongly, I ran to the bedroom to get the blood pressure cuff. Panic-stricken, I was shaking too badly to get a reading. On a second try my blood pressure was higher than it had ever been, and my pulse was around one-hundred-twenty beats per minute. Heart transplant recipients typically have high pulse rates and mine was usually around ninety beats per minute. My body and brain braced itself for another v-tach.

I could sense my muscles anticipating a shock from an I.C.D. I had to tell myself, "I don't have an I.C.D. I can't get shocked. My heart probably doesn't even know what v-tach is." My body didn't listen or didn't believe me. I began to sweat. I wanted to call the doctor, or 911, but realized that would be silly.

Luckily, Mom was visiting. She said I was having a panic attack and would be okay. She did the sweetest thing to comfort me: she led me through a creative visualization and then told me a bedtime story from my childhood. The sound of her voice was soothing, although it was hard to focus on what she was saying.

After fifteen minutes of feeling hot and sweaty from the panic attack, I began to calm down. Then I went through a cold and shaky phase, which lasted another fifteen minutes. Then, the longest portion of the experience was exhaustion accompanied by efforts to refocus on the reality of the present moment. It was a matter of trying to convince myself that nothing bad was going to happen. I needed to relax in the safety of my present circumstances.

I decided it must be time to deal with the post-traumatic stress of my experience.

Bravely deciding to face the truth of what happened to me seemed to lessen the anxiety. It wasn't easy. I did not like to talk about my condition. Even in the hospital, when doctors visited, I preferred they talk to Bob first. They would share with him the good or bad (usually bad) news first because then he could convey it to me in a more compassionate way.

So it was mostly through him that I learned about upcoming procedures and their successes (mostly failures) and whatever other tests and steps the doctors wanted to take. Bob was an excellent advocate on my behalf, and he assumed the role wholeheartedly. The downside was that I was able to avoid having to deal with my condition.

I forced myself to think about and retrace the steps to transplant. I revisited every detail: the loss of consciousness, the firings of the I.C.D., the unsuccessful weanings from the lidocaine, the failed ablations, the near-death experience, and the surgery. Finally I could think about these events calmly and without my mind drifting to other topics in pursuit of avoidance.

I also sensed I had to heal the relationships in my life. I thought about all those I had known and loved. Which relationships harbored ill feelings, unfinished business, or unresolved pain? Inwardly I spoke to each person who came to mind and listened for what they might have to tell me. I cannot say that I always heard replies in words. In some cases I felt ripples, like waves on a pond. When this occurred, I smoothed the ripples until I felt stillness within myself when I imagined the person in question.

Whenever possible or appropriate, I did the same outwardly. I phoned them. We talked. I apologized. In many cases outer communication could not occur, or I felt it best to keep the healing on my side of the karmic equation. As long as I honestly felt peace in my heart about each relationship, I knew the healing was completed.

Another approach I took was to examine my beliefs. This was the most revealing exercise I'd ever done. I began with a list of topics that meant something to me. They included: marriage, divorce, children, money, employment, career, success, my future, self-worth, my heart and the heart transplant, inner guidance, and spirituality.

I then would write: "Regarding [a subject from my list], I believe" and then I jotted down the first thing that came to my mind. Every one of these short, quick, spontaneous responses surprised me. I had no idea how little I knew about myself. Things that I thought I had issues with, I didn't. Things that I felt I was comfortable with and trusted needed work.

The two beliefs that were especially enlightening were about marriage and inner guidance. "Regarding marriage, I believe love will come in time." I did not want to hear that. I felt I had waited long enough to get married, and yet I also felt that ending my relationship with Bob was wrong. A conversation with my Aunt Vera set me straight. She said, "He just isn't ready." I had to learn to accept that and love unconditionally.

I've learned that every relationship has not two, but three partners—the third is God—or whatever you wish to call the All-knowing, All-powerful force that always gets Its way. If Bob and I got married, it would be in God's time.

One of the reasons I was anxious to get married stemmed from a premonition I had when I was a teen. I'd had a sudden knowing that my life's work would unfold when I was married. Since my first two marriages didn't work out, I wasn't sure why I felt so strongly that the premonition was still true. Nonetheless, I felt that once I was married, my problem of not having a career would solve itself.

The other belief that surprised me was: "Regarding my inner guidance, I have a lot yet to learn." I'd been conscientiously practicing divine guidance since I was sixteen. I thought I had a pretty good handle on it. After all, didn't the Light and Sound visit me every night? Time had its hand in this belief too. In time—and soon—I would learn a lot more about the capacity of inner guidance.

Meanwhile, my nightly inner experiences with the Light and Sound were islands in a sea of changes going on in my outer life. On the one hand, I was getting my health back; on the other hand, I still had a long way to go.

The train had come back into my awareness and a tunnel lay ahead.

As a heart transplant patient, I received regular heart biopsies which test for rejection. At first I got them weekly, and then progressively less often. In August 2005, at six months post-transplant, the results came back with the bad news. My body was rejecting my heart. The doctors would treat it by simply increasing my doses of anti-rejection meds. Then I'd have to go for another biopsy in a week rather than a month, as previously scheduled. The doctors made it seem as though rejection was no big deal. For me, it was huge.

When I heard the diagnosis, my first reaction was utter shock. How could the rejection have happened so suddenly without warning?

Ah, but I had been warned. I'd dreamt of being back on the train and heading into a tunnel. Plus, maybe the anxiety, the lightheadedness, and the skipping heartbeats were not just side effects of the meds.

I believe that everything that happens outwardly is a reflection of what goes on inwardly. Every significant event has a spiritual meaning or message or teaches us something about ourselves or life around us. What was the real message here? What was I really rejecting?

Did it have something to do with my nightly visits with the Light? In complete denial, I shut that thought immediately from my mind. Of course it didn't.

True, I hadn't had a conversation with my organs in several weeks. Were they resentful or feeling ignored? I didn't think so. I was feeling such harmony between and among my organs that I felt the cycle of consciously introducing them to each other was no longer necessary.

Still, I could not help feeling betrayed.

My body had let me down. It had rejected me.

My immune system was attacking my heart without provocation, permission, or warning. It was enacting a program of self-sabotage and self-destruction of the most heinous kind. Didn't my body realize it was essentially killing itself? Why?

On the one hand, I wanted the truth. On the other, I didn't want to hear it. So I pushed, I wished, and I willed myself to stop attacking and killing my heart. I explained the situation to the Spirit of my Immune System and reintroduced it to the Spirit of my Heart and begged them to cooperate.

In a less frantic moment, I asked my organ spirits if there was something I was rejecting in my outer life that was somehow mirrored within my body? If my organs knew and wanted to tell me, I was unable to hear them.

At my next biopsy, I learned that the rejection was over, and so I stopped asking what had gone wrong. My respite was short.

Five months later, I had another episode of rejection. This time I was ready to listen.

At a routine visit with my transplant team in January 2006, I reported light-headedness that was worse than ever. It would come in waves that took me to the edge of passing out. Unfortunately, my doctors did not have anything helpful to tell me. On the way out of their office, in the hospital foyer, I nearly lost consciousness. Bob wrapped his arm around my waist to keep me from falling, brought me back to the doctors' office and demanded they look into what was going wrong. They admitted me for observation.

The next day they did an angiogram and found my arteries were squeaky clean. What to do next?

"It's a shot in the dark," a doctor on my team told me, "but tomorrow, let's try a heart biopsy."

Tahdah! I was rejecting.

It was partly my fault. The immune-suppressing meds were making me feel nauseous, and I often skipped doses simply because I was feeling too sick to eat anything. (I was supposed to take the meds with food.) Heart transplant patients cannot do that without inviting trouble. The doctors lowered my dose to one we agreed might be more tolerable, and I had to promise to take it religiously.

The cure for the rejection was to give me rounds of anti-rejection meds intravenously for three days. While I rested in my hospital bed, the medicine was hooked up to the I.V. pole. When it began to drain, I could feel it run through my veins. Curious, I looked up at the bag of fluid and watched it drip rhythmically into the I.V. tube. The dripping lulled me into a deep relaxation, and a question arose from a deeper part of me than I was willing to explore before: What was the real reason I was here?

I slipped into a lucid dream-like experience that brought me to the Light. From within the Light, scenes emerged, and I learned something about my past lives.

First, I saw myself as a medical researcher in the nineteenth century. Somehow, my work in that lifetime set up the karmic circumstances for me to directly experience the fruits of my own research. I felt humbled by the fact that I was being healed by a medical philosophy I had once espoused in a past life.

To my amazement, I learned that this past life was not the only one in which I helped to develop new healing modalities. Millennia ago, in ancient China, I had experienced many lifetimes in which I experimented with acupuncture—both as the doctor and often as the slave upon whom the doctors practiced. I saw myself as an herbalist and midwife in Europe during the Middle Ages and being burned at the stake.

My lifetimes as an American Indian shaman held the most pleasant and vivid memories. The scenes that the Light revealed to me helped me recall knowledge and experiences. I knew the attributes and gifts of direction and how to invoke the power of the North, East, South, and West. I remembered an uncanny relationship with animals, plants, minerals, Mother Earth, the universe and stars, and all their unseen forces. I had an ability to draw out unwanted energies and invite healing ones into the body of my patients.

I had mystical abilities in that lifetime and was able to see the Light and foretell the future. In one prophetic vision, I'd seen rivers crowded with canoes that were powered without oars and traveled both up and down rivers. I had seen highways, yet at the time my mind could not translate the image of automobiles, and so I had seen canoes.

One more vision took me far back in time. I saw myself as a medicine woman living among a primitive tribe in southernmost South America. We would take yearly journeys to Antarctica to go hunting for seals and other aquatic game. In one scene, I was inside a den made of snow, tending the sick. Medicine back then was also energetic. Minerals, rocks, shells, feathers, soil samples, parts of plants, and other various natural items would be placed on or around the patient's body at just the right distances. In other words, I would make a mandala in a person's energy field. If the affliction involved someone else, an article belonging to that person was used. For reasons I cannot fathom today, the cures worked.

I was awakened when a nurse came to remove the empty I.V. bag.

I was glad she was too busy to chat because this adventure through my timeline had left me with a lot to think about. Foremost, I felt a sense of self-acceptance beginning to grow within me. I could no longer reject the truth of whom I had been, and I became more accepting of what my life's purpose might be. I also knew this would be my last experience of cardiac rejection.

Along a similar topic, my mind wandered to memories of one of my most fantastic dreams, which I'd had in the 1990s. In it, I was working off-planet in a huge, glass-domed botanical laboratory. My job was to develop a fruit that packed all the biochemicals needed for healing the ailments that one could expect on Earth. It would be seeded on Earth and cultivated there to provide a natural pharmacy for my people when they arrived on the planet.

Certainly this was the stuff of science fiction, yet the memories of working in that laboratory were as real to me as those of my microbiology lab in college.

When I awoke from the dream, I had an instant knowing of various ways the fruit's juice could be used as a home remedy. I wrote a preliminary list of about twenty-one ways and presented my idea to a publisher. They immediately agreed to work with me. In 1999, we published *53 Ways to Use Noni Fruit Juice for Your Better Health*. A year or two later, I added more ideas and we released *76 Ways to Use Noni*.

Had these dreams and lucid experiences contained but a kernel of truth, it meant I had an affinity with the healing arts. It was a theme that ran though many of my lifetimes on Earth and elsewhere. By 2006, my work with noni and other liquid nutritional supplements had ended, so I doubted I'd be pursuing them anymore. The other experience I'd had with the healing arts in this lifetime involved gemstones. I did not want to get involved with gemstones again, and even if I did, I had no clue how it could happen.

In the weeks that followed this final rejection, my nightly soirees into the Light began to shift. Although I did not consciously remember any specific instruction just yet, my attitude about working with gemstones must have been softening.

A few months later, during an evening soiree with the Light, I heard an inner voice say, "You have an unfulfilled contract with David." Then during my waking hours, feelings that I still owed David information on gemstones surfaced, even as I tried to ignore them. They quite literally badgered me inwardly.

Bob was strongly against me working with David. He truly believed it was wrong to be in business with an ex-spouse. Looking back, I sensed he was picking up on the wrongness of me working for anyone except myself. My destiny with Gemstone Therapy could not be fulfilled sailing on anyone else's ship. Until I could set out by myself, which was not even a thought at that time, I needed to complete my karma with David.

In the spring of 2006, the inner pressure to complete that contract became unbearable. On the one hand, I wanted to respect Bob's feelings about not getting re-involved with David. On the other, I desperately needed work. The royalties from my books on liquid nutritional supplements, which had supported me during my heart failure, were tapering off. Because of my health, I was unable to work outside the home, and I did not have enough social security to draw benefits. I had to find something I could do, and tried a few things unsuccessfully.

Finally, I telephoned David. This in itself wasn't unusual because we had remained in contact during my illness. He would regularly call and ask how I was doing. After all, I was the mother of our three children, and he was genuinely concerned.

In this conversation, after we talked about the kids, I asked him if he would be interested in me researching some new gemstones for his company. This time, however, I would not channel the gemstone guardians. Instead, I would consciously visit them and the doctors involved with Gemstone Therapy on the inner planes and interview them directly. Or I would visit the Great Library and get the information there. I was not sure how I knew I could do this. I just knew.

To my surprise, David told me he had already been thinking of the idea, and so we struck an agreement. He would send me gemstone samples, and I would record my inner-world experiences with them. The recordings would be transcribed and then he and others on the editorial team would ask questions about what I'd learned so far, and I would go back to find the answers.

Soon after the agreement was made, my nightly visits with the Light took shape and my understanding of the capacity of inner guidance exploded. From within the Light, a man appeared, who said he was a Gemstone Therapy teacher. He suggested I call him Dr. Ay because his true name was an impossible string of vowels that was too foreign to my earthly ear. "Ay" was the first syllable in that sequence.

Dr. Ay stood about nine feet tall and always wore white. He invited me to his office. So I left my body behind and followed him there. The room was spacious, white, somewhat round, and in the center, furnished with two white rectangular benches-with-backs that proved to be more comfortable than they looked. A wall of windows on the west side of the room revealed our location high in the mountains. The view was stunning. Snow-capped peaks loomed as far as the eye could see. I suspected this was northern Tibet and eventually learned his office was located in a spiritual city there.

My visits to his office became routine. Each time, I would sit on one bench and he would sit across from me on the other. Dr. Ay taught me about the gemstones by telepathic communication and by demonstrations using a "library box." This was a foot-wide opaque white cube that sat on a square white table between us. When Dr. Ay wanted to demonstrate a concept, he would activate the library box, and a holographic image of what he wanted to show me would appear projected above it. Sometimes the images were small, other times, life-sized.

With the library box, I learned everything from human energetic anatomy to the way energy moves through gemstones. I saw the energy pictures of diseases and the effects of gemstone treatments on the body, chakras, and aura. Seeing these images helped me to also identify energetic anomalies in myself and others and how to correct them using the gems.

At times we would also visit what reminded me of a surgical viewing theater where we would watch Gemstone Therapy taking place. While sitting behind a special screen, we could witness, in living color, the energetic shifts happening in the patient being treated.

While I had fought bitterly with myself to avoid stepping back into the world of gemstones, once I did, I remembered how much I loved it. No longer did I need to wait for bedtime to dip into the Light. I could go to the inner libraries when I felt calm, focused, and grateful. Now that my heart was open to receiving the information about Gemstone Therapy, the information was given to me and it poured forth prolifically.

Still, I was not following my inner blueprints perfectly enough, and I was about to discover the consequences.

23

MY LIFE FALLS APART

*O*ne afternoon in the autumn of 2007, I was down on my knees cleaning the wood floors in our kitchen. I didn't like the smell of the citrus wood cleaner, so it was an unpleasant chore. Bob was downstairs in the "man-cave" he had built for himself in the basement.

Bob has a big voice, so I knew he was on the phone. It sounded as though he was talking to a long-time friend, which he often did, and I paid no attention.

Suddenly, either Bob began to speak more loudly, or my hearing improved exponentially, or the kitchen floors became thinner, because I thought I heard him say, "I'm planning to leave."

I must have heard wrong.

I was sure I did.

I needed to hear more. My body began to shake as the details were confided over the phone. I heard only bits and pieces of the conversation.

"She's pushing me out." I heard him say, "The relationship isn't working for me anymore."

I knew that eavesdropping is a form of encroachment, and I felt awful for doing it. Here I was, with my ear to the floor, making myself doubly sick inhaling citrus solvent. Literally, I had lowered myself.

"...No... I haven't told Isa yet... I've told one other person... and now you."

I felt as though a train had hit me. Or that some inner cork had been pulled and all my energy was draining out. While I knew Bob was not content with our relationship, I never expected it to actually end. Bob had been my rock, care-giver, and supporter. More than that, I thought we were meant for each other. It made no sense for us to be apart.

When the conversation was over, I met Bob in the kitchen.

"Do you have anything to tell me?" I stood with my arms folded, leaning against the kitchen sink. I needed all the support I could get.

Bob grabbed the tea kettle. "I was downstairs talking to Steve."

I stared at the back of his head and waited for a better answer while he made the tea. I didn't get one. With tea in hand, he retreated to the living room.

I withdrew to my bed, which had always been a place of comfort. Too restless to relax, I got back up and went outside for a walk. The autumn air felt especially cold, and the leafless trees looked as stripped of life as I myself felt. I went inside, sat at my desk, and tried to tidy up. Nothing worked to ease the separation anxiety.

I had to confront him.

He was sitting in the living room, which showcased his impressive collection of audio equipment. He had made the room cozy with furniture he had refinished himself, oriental rugs, plants, and choice pieces of my free-form crochet artwork. It was my favorite room in the house.

I brought some yarn and a crochet hook with me and sat down on the armchair beside the fireplace. I often crocheted while we watched television or listened to music.

This time, I could hardly work the yarn. My fingers would not stop shaking, my insides felt knotted, and my throat was one big lump. I didn't know if my angst was visible or if Bob even cared. "Can we talk?" I kept my focus on my crocheting.

"Sure." He kept his attention on a record album he was looking at.

"What's going on?"

"Just playing with my stereo equipment." He had a small pile of vinyl laying on the coffee table.

"I know you aren't happy here."

"I've told you a million times I'm not comfortable with a woman working for her ex-husband. It just isn't right. Ask anyone, and they'll tell you the same thing. Maybe your friends will say there's nothing wrong with it. I'm old-fashioned. I think it's wrong."

Yes, Bob had warned me about that very often. I loved Bob. I loved working with the gemstones too. Besides, I had no other source of income.

"You always had a choice," he said. "Our relationship or the gemstones. You made your choice, so I made mine." He went over to his record rack and pulled out a few more albums.

He was right. I had been taking him and our relationship for granted. I had made my work priority and ignored his feelings. I had hoped he would find a way to reconcile them. I had hoped he would change.

"I don't want to give up the relationship," I said.

"You should have made that decision a long time ago."

Bob decided to leave during the Christmas holiday. My dad and his wife, Fenella, were sensitive to my situation and gifted me enough money to bring me and my two youngest children to Oregon to celebrate Christmas with my eldest three children. At least I wouldn't have to be there when Bob moved out.

We were welcomed to stay with David and his wife and enjoyed a truly magical holiday. I had all five of my children together at once—parents will know how special that is. Christmas morning the snow began to fall, and the world was beautiful. I felt that Nature was telling me this was a purification. If so, it was a painful one.

Indeed, my emotions were making my energies flighty and uncontrollable. I felt disconnected from my body and could not relax or fall asleep. I was not taking the breakup well at all.

"Try wearing Onyx," someone suggested. "It will help you feel more grounded."

For some reason, it was difficult for me to wear the Onyx. This reminded me of another reason I had previously left the world of gemstones. I felt hypocritical in that I promoted therapeutic gemstone necklaces yet could not wear them myself. I would try, but after an hour or so I'd have to take them off.

Later on, when I found out about symbiotic gemstones, I would understand why this was so. The presence of symbiotic stones in a necklace can make a huge difference in the way a wearer receives the gemstone energies. When Onyx is strung with Ruby, I am able to wear the necklace all day long.

One night during that Christmas holiday, my eldest two daughters took me to a bar where a hip-hop band was playing. I danced for hours. This was the first sweet relief that I felt. I had forgotten how much I loved to dance. Moving my body to the music released the tension and got my energies flowing once again. I could not believe how I'd lost my focus. Over the past few weeks, I had taken my new heart for granted. Dancing reminded me that I was alive. My life was full of promise and could be full of love again too.

Despite this island of happiness, the despondency persisted.

By the time I got back home after the New Year, I had no more tears left to cry. I felt like a tree whose leaves and bark had been stripped by a hurricane. My heart felt incapable of giving love or receiving it. This was the darkest winter of my life. The Light had gone out of reach and become invisible to me. I imagined its presence—I knew it was there—but my means of contact no longer worked.

I had never felt so alone.

Life became a matter of going through the mechanical motions instilled by years of habit. I got up, worked at my computer, did my chores, and went to bed. I hardly ate, and I hardly slept. I felt I could no longer live in my house and decided to sell. The memories of Bob there were too many. I couldn't wait to move on and get this horrible chapter of my life behind me.

My single joy was caring for my tropical fish. Before I left for Oregon that Christmas, I had a dream about a certain golden-yellow tropical fish.

"I'm Gazebo," the fish said in the dream. "Find me and I will show you love."

How nice, I thought. *I'll get some fish for pets.* I'd heard pets could aid the grieving process.

I went to two different stores, where none of the fish stood out. I told AriaRay and Kellan about the dream, and together we went to another pet store to see if Gazebo was there. We searched through all the tanks. When we looked at the tank of Candy Parrot Cichlids, they looked back at us with what looked like conscious awareness. I mentioned this to the store owner.

He laughed and agreed, "They are intelligent fish."

Not surprisingly, among them, we found Gazebo. She held our attention the longest, and I'm sure I felt a heart connection between us, too.

I purchased a 55-gallon tank, somewhat hesitantly, because

it was my full intention to pack up the house and move as soon as I possibly could. Moving a large fish tank would make the job all the more complicated. Oh well. I was following one nudge at a time. It was all I could do.

I also adopted a few smaller fish and a friend for Gazebo, another Parrot Cichlid, whom we named Bella. The first day in the tank, Gazebo came up to my fingers when I held food for her. Bella stayed at the bottom of the tank. This scenario replayed for three days and I was getting worried that Bella was not eating. Maybe he was feeling the deep despondency, as I was, of having had your world completely rearranged. This I could totally relate to.

On the fourth day, I was feeding the fish and feeling terribly low and hopeless. In a moment of doubt and desperation I said aloud, "Show me love."

I thought I had been talking to God. But Gazebo responded as though she had heard me. Suddenly, she stopped eating. Have you ever seen a fish stop feeding once it has started? I never had. So this alone was unusual. Then came the miraculous: Gazebo swam to the bottom of the tank where Bella was hiding. She nudged him relentlessly until he swam up to the food I was holding. When he finally started to eat, then she did too.

Gazebo taught me that miracles are possible. Love is real— and it exists even among tropical fish. My heart began to heal.

One morning soon after, I sat down in my office, which Bob had wallpapered years before with a paper that had a green leaf print. I always felt surrounded by the abundance of nature in this room. I opened my email and found one from him.

I held my finger over the delete button.

I looked over at my fish tank, which stood a mere three feet from my desk. Gazebo and Bella were happily swimming together.

I opened the email. Bob wanted to talk.

We agreed to meet a few days later for tea.

I waited for him in a crowded diner. The sound of other peoples' voices made me feel comfortably inconspicuous. As soon as Bob arrived, I felt a little better. As soon as we started talking about the weather and how our families were doing, the agony eased even more.

We escaped from the small talk.

"You know, I felt as though you were pushing me away ever since you began working for your ex-husband."

"I wasn't."

"But that's how I felt."

The waitress arrived with our order. I sipped the tea and nibbled at some toast.

"Then, when you learned our relationship was over," he said, "I couldn't understand why you fell apart. I thought you'd be glad. Relieved to move on with the gemstones without me holding you back."

I noticed Bob wasn't eating much either.

"You really had no idea how much I loved you?" I asked. The past tense felt like a wall of protection.

"When I finished loading my stuff into the truck and walked out your door for the last time," Bob said, "I knew I was leaving my life behind. But I felt cornered. Like there was no room for me in our relationship. I needed to escape."

"I love working with the gemstones."

"I know."

Bob played with his teacup, as though trying to make it fit into the grooves on the saucer. "What I don't know," he paused, "is if there is any hope that you and I could get back together?"

My insides relaxed for the first time in months.

He asked, "It would be nice if, maybe, we could talk again or at least share email?"

I gobbled down the toast, suddenly feeling famished.

As the warmth of spring coaxed buds from the branches of seemingly lifeless trees, it brought back life to me and to our relationship.

That June, 2008, with the leaves flush with summer warmth, Bob and I went to Maine. After dinner, we took a walk beside the sea. The sun was beginning to paint the clouds with sunset colors. We turned onto the wooden walkway to Marshall Point lighthouse. We leaned on the railing to watch the sky, breathe in the fresh ocean air, and listen to the gulls.

Bob fumbled for something in his pocket. I wouldn't have noticed, except that he also took my hand in his and held it firmly. He took out what he'd been searching for and held between us an Aquamarine and Diamond ring.

"Isabelle, will you marry me?"

The blue of his eyes, the blue of the Aquamarine, and the blue of the water fused in my brain. I felt speechless. I knew my silence was making him uncomfortable. Why wasn't I answering him? Was it because I was struck by disbelief that after dating for eight years I was finally getting the proposal I had always wanted? Was it because the turn of events seemed nothing short of miraculous? Or was I doubting that Bob was really ready to have a relationship that included the gemstones?

I didn't mean to make him suffer. Poor guy, I could practically see him begin to sweat. When his words registered in both my mind and heart, I blurted out my answer.

"Yes!"

We were married in November 2008.

Later, when I asked Bob how he was finally able to accept both me and my work, he simply said, "I let it go." He reminded me that it wasn't the gemstones themselves he had issue with, it was a feeling that he couldn't share me with my ex-husband—even if it was just in business. "Besides," he said, "I felt my life belonged with you."

Bob and I are aware of a past life we shared in Europe in the aftermath of World War II. By piecing our memories together, the reason for our relationship today has unfolded.

I was a Frenchwoman and a member of the resistance. I was imprisoned with others and nearly starved to death in a dank underground cellar. When the fighting ended we were abandoned, as the soldiers who fed us either fled or were killed or captured. A vivid memory of mine is the silhouette of a soldier framed by the sunlight that poured through the door when he unlocked it.

Bob remembers being an Allied soldier in World War II, rescuing a nearly lifeless woman, and the instant connection they shared. It was love at first sight—a recognition between two Souls who had shared many previous lifetimes together. He carried me to freedom and made sure I got the medical attention I needed. Sadly, I was too far gone, and died in his arms.

This lifetime imprinted upon Bob the need to take care of me as best he could—to keep me alive. Quite literally, he has done so. Awareness of this past life has also imprinted on me the need to accept the care. Not only is it a karmic contract, it is a demonstration of love, in both directions. Receiving love is also an act of love.

In making our marriage commitment, things between us improved. In order to make the relationship work, we both let go of certain things and took responsibility for others. Moreover, our love deepened. In each other we have found not only someone whom we can love—but also, more importantly, someone who will receive our love. That's the rarest. Not once when I have tried to give Bob affection has he refused me and vice versa. We sense each other's rhythms, respect each other's needs, and go out of our way to do kind things for each other. We give and receive, back and forth.

In this world of opposites in which we live, I've come to realize that you cannot truly appreciate health until you lose it. You cannot know happiness until you know despair, and you cannot love truly until love has been taken away.

Bob and I each gained freedom when we forgave each other. Doing so was one of the best decisions I've ever made. Now I was faced with one of the biggest.

24

THE DAM BURSTS

*W*hen Bob and I started mending our relationship, the light that visited me at night returned. It was sweet relief to be bathing in it once again.

After our wedding, something shifted significantly. It was an inner feeling of something being different, but I couldn't define what it was. It manifested in my feeling increasingly guilty about writing anonymously about the therapeutic benefits of gemstones. Why couldn't I go public? What was I afraid of?

The conflict hounded me for weeks.

In early January 2009, I finally admitted to myself the truth: I did not want to be ostracized by my family, friends, or those on my spiritual path. I wanted the freedom to teach and talk about Gemstone Therapy and at the same time continue with the volunteer work I was doing at our temple. Today, I cannot tell you why I ever thought these activities would be mutually exclusive. For whatever reason, the fear felt real.

I discovered a seed cause of my problem. I realized that the "very spiritual" woman who had given me the condescending look so many years ago was not so spiritual after all. If she had been the high being I thought she was, then she would not have sent me such bad vibrations—no matter what I was doing.

219

After all, my spiritual guides have always stuck by me, even when I've made the most stupid decisions. They were even there when I chose to channel. They love me unconditionally—like Bob now did. In contrast, this woman was full of judgment, and I let her affect me. Finally, her opinion no longer mattered. She fell from the pedestal I had put her on.

I felt instant relief.

Next, I had to clear my conscience with my family.

"Did you know your mom is weird?" I said to Kellan and AriaRay. We were making cupcakes, as we did most weekends. I got out the ingredients, and they measured and mixed. I kept my tone as casual as I could. "I'm as weird as it gets. But I love you anyway, and I know you love me anyway."

"We know that," AriaRay said. "Do we have organic sugar?"

I grabbed it from the pantry. "You know I'm weird?"

"I don't think you're weird," AriaRay said. "Kellan, stop making a mess with the flour."

She had spilled some on the countertop.

"Everyone is weird," Kellan said, fully focused on sifting the flour into the measuring cup. "Get over it."

The door of my invisible cage flung open.

With my fears finally in perspective, I no longer cared if people thought I was crazy, or doing something they thought was wrong. I had been accused of dabbling in the psychic worlds, when I should have my attention on the highest spiritual planes. I didn't think I was crazy, or doing anything psychic—certainly not any more than anyone else who studied and applied alternative healing methods.

The truth was that I loved working with gemstones. I had some unexplainable affinity with them. The thought of teaching the work to others who also loved gems made my heart burst with joy. I couldn't contain it any longer.

I phoned David and asked him to include my name as "gemstone researcher" on his website, underneath the credits for editor and webmaster. I also offered to begin training his customers via teleseminars and workshops. I wanted to develop Gemstone Therapy protocols for target areas, chakras, systems, and color rays so that when a client came in for help, there would be a logical and consistent approach to meeting the person's concerns.

"I cannot do that," David said. He explained that it was his intention all along to keep my identity anonymous. He could not risk the possibility that I might leave again as I had done at our divorce. Back then, in 1992, the business nearly did not survive the loss.

I had no idea.

I have always appreciated David's desire to preserve and protect the business. Still, he insisted that as long as I was working for him, I would remain in the background. All along, I had believed David was patiently waiting for me to be okay with going public, so that we could step forward in a much bigger way. The misunderstanding hurt.

In the end, this was just as well because I was able to draw a clear dividing line between my work with his company and the projects I wanted to pursue.

The decision to let go of anonymity was a huge turning point for me. My nightly forays into the Light took on a different quality. Although I do not remember what was going on, the next three nights were intensive. Parts of me beyond my conscious awareness were working very hard—to the point that I felt spiritually exhausted by the time I fell asleep. I suspect I was being tested as to whether or not I could go the distance.

I knew I had passed the tests when, on the fourth night, I barely got into bed when the Light was there as though waiting for me. I was met by a deluge of creativity, as though a dam

221

had burst. While my inner vision was flooded with Light, my head became filled with knowledge about circular configurations of single gemstone spheres. These configurations, or gemstone mandalas, were called "gemandalas."

I turned on my bedside lamp, got out a notebook, and started drawing geometrical designs that consisted of various gems. Each gemandala had a specific healing purpose. I was amazed at the range of possibilities. There could be a gemandala that matched the frequency picture of any manifestation of ill health or imbalance—even as it varied among person to person—whether its origin was physical, emotional, or mental.

I transported myself to Dr. Ay's office. I couldn't wait to ask, "What can you tell me about gemandalas?"

"Well, it's about time," he teased.

"Have you been waiting for me?"

Dr. Ay stood up. "Come with me," he said.

I was reminded how very tall he was. Nearly twice my height. He led me out of his office and into a curved hallway that was completely white and perfectly clean. I noticed the faint scent of fresh flowers. We entered a room that looked like a small amphitheater. The floor of the room consisted of steps that led to a treatment table in the center, upon which a woman was lying down covered by a thin pale-blue blanket. Someone stood behind her, organizing gemstone necklaces, trays of gemstone spheres, and bottles of liquid on a long, narrow table.

"I would like you to observe a Gemstone Therapy session," Dr. Ay said in a hushed voice. "The client is a woman who recently moved to a new town and developed a persistent skin rash."

The practitioner who worked on her began by draping a series of necklaces over his client's body.

Dr. Ay whispered, "One of the first steps in any Gemstone Therapy session is to use certain gemstone necklaces that promote balance in the five elements. These are water, wood, fire, earth, and metal. Every process and function of every cell, organ, and aspect of the body are driven and described by these elements. The gems awaken the body to its five-element processes and relationships so that the body can begin to self-correct any fundamental imbalances that may exist."

The practitioner then wrapped a necklace around a wooden wand and applied it in the client's aura using circle-like movements.

"He is performing another initial gemstone application, this time, to clear unwanted energies that may have collected in the subject's aura."

As he did, the light around the client grew brighter.

"Now he is going to build a gemandala. You'll have to step closer to see."

"Is that okay?"

"Yes. The client has already given us permission to observe the session."

I walked down the steps up to the treatment table in the center of the room and watched. The practitioner attached small, 4-to-6-millimeter round gemstones to a beeswax-covered disk that was attached to a wooden rod. One by one, new gems were put in place until, at some point, the practitioner must have felt the arrangement was complete.

He then held the rod with the gems facing his client's body and moved it in circles, spirals, and various other ways. As he did, we could see the effects the gems were having on the aura around the client as well as on the energies that comprised her body. Some areas were like a sponge, eagerly absorbing the gemstones' energies as though filling deficiencies in her life-energy. Other areas, where energy seemed tight and congested, were relieved. Ripples in the woman's energies, which corresponded to unwanted patterns, were smoothed. Where negative, unwanted energies had collected, they were corralled and then dissipated.

I wondered if the movements the practitioner used were random.

"Each movement has a reason and a purpose," Dr. Ay explained. "When you understand why a certain movement is performed over a certain area, you can gain insight into what's going on energetically in that area."

"How does the practitioner know what movements to use?"

"He doesn't," Dr. Ay said. "He simply follows the energy of his client's body."

I must have looked doubtful.

Dr. Ay explained, "Gemstones have an affinity with the body's energy, and the body recognizes gemstone energies. When you bring gems into the aura, the body's energy field will begin to move them in archetypical ways. A practitioner simply follows these movements to give the body the gemstone energies exactly how and where they are needed."

I would eventually document twenty-seven of these movements, including the circles and spirals we were watching now.

We listened as the practitioner described the gemandala he was using to his client.

"The central gemstone in this mandala is Yellow Sapphire," he explained to her. "Around it we have three Rose Quartz and three Picture Jasper in a circle. The presence of the Yellow Sapphire suggests that the rash is due to a difficulty of the eliminatory processes in the skin. The Rose Quartz tells us the difficulty involves releasing certain emotions. And the Picture Jasper suggests that the emotions in question are those involved with your struggle to adapt to your new environment."

"That makes sense," she said. "It has been a struggle. And the rash only appeared after I moved."

"The gemandala suggests you may have pent up emotions about your recent change of jobs. These emotions are interfering with a healthy release of toxins, and so the physical ailment manifested."

The woman nodded and confirmed that what he said was correct. The light of awareness crossed her face as she now had something definitive to think about and process.

"All gemandalas can be interpreted this way," Dr. Ay said.

"How did he know which gems to use?" I asked.

"This is the beauty of Gemstone Therapy," he said with a grin. "The gemstones are chosen not by the practitioner—but by client's own intelligence centers. The practitioner uses any number of different ways to determine those choices. Based on the gemstones chosen, we can learn a great deal about what is going on energetically behind the scenes of a condition."

"Do all conditions have energetic causes?"

"Most do," he replied. "Disharmony can originate at any level of manifestation. These levels are: atomic, molecular, cellular, organ, system, whole body, and whole being. The whole-body level is further divided into the physical, supraphysical, emotional, causal, and mental bodies."

His mention of levels of manifestation rang a bell. I'd heard that term before.

He continued, "Unless a disharmony is resolved at the level of manifestation where it originated, no amount of physical treatment will cure. Symptoms may pass—for a while—but they will return sooner or later. Symptoms are the body's way of communicating inner disharmony. Gemstone energies can balance disharmony in a way that also teaches and enlightens. Gemstone energies are not erasers; they're instructors. Let's take an even closer look at the gemandala chosen for this woman's skin rash."

I learned that the properties of the gemstones in the geman-dala—as well as the geometry and numerologies involved—all contributed special meaning and intent.

"Because the gems appeared in threes," Dr. Ay said, "the mandala can support the individual through the changes she wants to make. Because the gems formed a hexagon around the central gemstone, we know this condition is helping the woman toward self-mastery. This means she would have to put forth extra effort in her life in general to overcome her specific situation. The lessons she learns in resolving the skin rash will serve in other areas of her spiritual unfoldment too."

He continued, "Applying the gemandala to the aura associated with the afflicted area will help release the emotions stuck there, vitalize the skin and its eliminatory processes, and help this woman come to harmony with her present circumstances."

By the end of the session, the woman's inflamed skin appeared more pink than red. It no longer radiated angry energies. The client herself appeared calm and also eager to step back into her life with a new attitude.

My mind burst with the possibilities.

One of my concerns about Gemstone Therapy had been the investment involved. While many people are blessed to be able to purchase one or more necklaces, the modality could not go mainstream unless it became affordable. However, only a relatively small investment would be required to build a practice that focused on making and applying gemandalas.

Dr. Ay told me that only eight of each kind of gem were required. Any more would be impractical for this application. Someone with a collection of thirty or so different gemstone spheres could make a gemandala to address almost any intention.

"In a Gemstone Therapy session," Dr. Ay said, "you make gemandalas that are tailored for your client. Imagine gemandalas that

226

have a universal appeal. Imagine gemandalas that could benefit a wide population."

"That would be wonderful," I said, and then thought of an objection. "Not everyone has the dexterity to work with the stones. Besides, how many people would actually take the time to self-apply the gemandalas in the aura long enough to make a difference?"

"There is another way."

We left the therapy viewing room, and I followed him, wondering what he could have possibly meant. We returned to his office.

"Have a seat," he said and turned on the library box.

An image was projected above the box of a silvery tray with glass bottles of liquids.

I recognized them immediately. They were the decanters that Hahn once used, so many years ago, to heal David's leg!

"You could make these," he said.

"With sunlight?" I knew this was how gemstone elixirs were made. In my experience, this method did not hold the gemstone energies very long. I wondered if he knew a trick to improve their shelf life.

"There is a way that is far more effective."

I picked up on what he was hinting at and started feeling electrified with inspiration. If I could make liquids like this, then they would be even more affordable than a collection of gemstone spheres. They would be a far more practical way to bring Gemstone Therapy to the world.

My excitement drew me back to my bedroom. I had so much to think about!

I was holding a dream: of Gemstone Therapy becoming a mainstream world-wide modality, and the real possibility that this dream could come true.

Of course, the information I'd learned brought up a boat-load of curiosities. What gemandalas to start with? What types of products could be made? What would I call them, and most critically, how would I make them?

I knew the answers would come, and they did.

25

GEMSTONE FORMULAS ARE BORN

*D*uring the spring and summer of 2009, I was given information as fast as I could write it down. I would go to bed, step into the light, and write for a few hours every night. Then I'd try to get some sleep to keep my health in balance.

The inner-world members of my team were generously helpful. They gave me discourses on energetics and the technologies I would need to learn in order to build the device that would transfer the gemandala energies into alcohol. It would be called a "Gemstone Energy Field Imprinting device," or G.E.F.I.

I have a friend who collects alternative energy healing devices and enlisted his help to build a crucial part. I also asked my dad for help. He's a world-class engineer and was able to verify and give feedback on the principles I was learning inwardly (although I didn't tell him about that). At the time, nobody knew.

I've learned the hard way to keep quiet about what I'm developing. The process of manifesting something new is so fragile that anyone's doubts or negative thinking can shut down momentum and enthusiasm. I knew I needed to keep what I was learning to myself until it manifested physically. Then it couldn't be thwarted.

Soon enough I was given the first three formulas that we would release: Energy Clearing, Electro-magnetic Radiation Clearing, and

Core Alignment. They would be made using complex gemstone mandalas that contained as many as a hundred gemstones. The energies of the gemstones were imparted into organic grape alcohol, mixed with water, and then poured into spray bottles.

Spraying the aura brought the gemstone energies to the subtle bodies and the energetic counterparts of physical areas. There, the subtle-body intelligences would make pathways that could move the gemstone energies wherever they were needed most.

At times, I was so busy working for David's company during the day and manifesting the gem formulas in the evenings that I fell asleep as soon as my head hit the pillow. I'd miss a night in the Light. Sometimes, I'd go to bed, all ready with notebook in hand, and then nothing. I'd just fall asleep. Or, I'd wake up in the middle of the night with new information. Ventures into the Light came with the responsibility of recording what I learned. This could mean getting up from the warm, cozy blankets to grab a pen and notebook, and if Bob was in bed, as quietly as possible jotting down notes—in the dark—so not to wake him.

The creative process was fun, enlivening, and really exciting. It was also easy in that it was all taking place under the cloak of silence. I didn't have to summon the courage to share it, explain it, or tell anyone about it.

In early 2009, David was in Costa Rica and out of touch by phone or internet. Inwardly I felt tension building between us. I sensed our business relationship coming to a close. When in February I received an email from one of his staff asking me to return to his company all the gemstones I had been using, I knew my premonitions were correct.

At first, the request felt like a setback. Then I realized what a blessing it was. It meant that I would be using only my own gemstones to make the gemandalas. This was extremely important to the integrity of what I was doing. The gemandalas would be truly my own. It also got me started rebuilding relationships with previous suppliers of therapeutic-quality gemstones as well as finding others on my own.

When David returned to the United States in June, 2009, he called and formally dismissed me from his employ. It can be devastating to be fired from a job you love, especially when you have no other source of income. On the other hand, I instinctively knew that in order to end our karmic involvement, I could not quit or leave. He had to let me go. Now that he did, I could move forward full-time with my own gemstone business.

I was free. Scared, but free.

Now, nothing held me back but my own fears. It was one thing to learn this new information; it was quite another to share it with others. Spurring me forward was basic financial need. Thankfully Mom, and my brother, Paul, and his wife, Kathy, came to my aid, and Dad and his wife helped with the mortgage. Otherwise foreclosure was a real possibility.

All I could do was identify a step that felt right, take it, and then look for the next one. This is how I had kept moving forward when I was sick. The process worked for my business too.

On the one hand, I had everything to lose, on the other, nothing. After all, I had almost lost my life. That put everything else into proper perspective.

Bob's attitude about money was a source of comfort. When I discussed my situation, he'd say, "I'd be happy living in a tent." I knew I would be, too. He has taught me that happiness and money have nothing to do with each other.

That summer I was given the name of my new business. It would be called "GEMFormulas," which stood for Gemstone Energy Medicine Formulas. On July 17, 2009, an attorney completed the paperwork.

While the inner guidance continued, I did everything I could outwardly. I handled every detail of launching a company that I could think of and found the creative process both enjoyable and personally challenging.

I had so much to learn!

I had to teach myself how to build and maintain our website, film and edit instructional videos, and design workflows for stringing necklaces, taking orders, and keeping track of inventory. Having no prior business experience, I had no idea if I was doing the right thing. I felt pressed against my inner edge, and then stretched, pressed and stretched, in a constant effort toward self-expansion.

"How on Earth am I going to handle this?" I'd say when faced with each new challenge. Then the answer would come.

It was the Spirit of my Abdomen who taught me a lesson about courage. To explain how it happened, let me tell you about my heart biopsies. My first one took place in the hospital in February 2005, a week after the transplant. Nobody told me what to expect. They wheeled me into the procedure room on a gurney, and I braced myself to meet the unknown. To start, the doctor numbed the left side of my neck, and then inserted a catheter into my jugular vein. Guided by an x-ray machine, whose images were visible from a television monitor hanging from the ceiling, he threaded a wire into the catheter, through the vein, and into my heart.

The wire had a scissors-like handle on one end and pinchers on the other, which would bite off a small chunk of heart tissue. Whenever a sample was taken, my heart skipped a beat, and my body jerked.

"Does everyone feel it?" I asked.

"Not everyone."

Sometimes I think I am way too sensitive for my own good.

Biopsies are no big deal for most people. For me, they were unpleasant at best. After my fourth biopsy, in March, 2005, it seemed as though the doctor spent half an hour trying to push the catheter into my neck without success. Finally I asked him to stop.

He didn't.

"Let's do this another day."

He persisted.

"She asked you to stop," the attending nurse said.

Finally, he gave up. The left side of my neck would swell to the size of a grapefruit.

They gave me a sedative to ease my discomfort and repeated the procedure through the vein on the right side of my neck. This went smoothly. An ultrasound on my left jugular vein revealed a blood clot, which was the reason they were unable to insert the catheter.

Afterwards, while we sat with my cardiologist in her office, I found out the unpleasant ramifications of having a blood clot. I would have to go on blood thinning medicine for a few months until the clot went away. I had two more biopsies scheduled in the next month, so I could not go on an oral blood thinner. It would remain in my system too long and put me at risk for uncontrolled bleeding at my next biopsy.

She explained, "You'll have to use a different type of blood thinner, which metabolizes more quickly out of your system. You'll administer it by giving yourself a shot twice a day in your abdomen."

"What?" I could not believe my ears.

She repeated the instructions.

"With a needle?"

"Yes."

"In my belly?"

I hate, hate, hate needles.

The assignment pressed me against the edge of my emotional envelope. All the peace I had been enjoying by being home from the hospital and on a healing track evaporated. The thought of giving myself a shot was bad enough—having to do it in the stomach was so high on my queasy scale that I just could not deal with it.

At that time, I had hardly any fat on my stomach, and the needle had to be inserted subcutaneously. I worried I wouldn't have enough room on my stomach for two shots a day for the next thirty days. If this was a test of my self-control and perseverance, I did not think I was going to pass.

My eyes leaked saltwater for the next few hours. I had not cried since I'd come home from the hospital a few weeks earlier and had to admit the emotional release felt good.

"We can do this," the Spirit of my Abdomen assured me. "There's a bigger picture here."

"Bob told me that, back when my heart first failed."

"There's a bigger picture here," Spirit of my Abdomen repeated.

"What is it?"

"You have to learn courage."

"Why?"

"Because."

The Spirit of my Abdomen suggested I give myself a shot in the early morning, first thing, before I was awake enough to think about it, and the second one sometime around dinner so I could get it over with before the nightfall when I might start procrastinating.

Whenever I was about to insert the needle, I warned the Spirit of my Abdomen. "Here it comes," I'd say.

One evening she spoke up loud and clear: "There's got to be another way."

"I thought we were learning courage?"

I had a growing collection of quarter-inch bruises across my midsection. One for each injection.

"There's got to be another way."

I called my nurse. "If the injection needs to be subcutaneous, can I use the fatty tissue on my buttocks instead?"

"Yes, that would be fine."

Whew, what a blessing. That was so much easier to handle emotionally.

The experience taught me courage. When a step appears— and you know you have to take it—you just take it. It also taught me to trust time. Soon enough, this part of my journey ended as did all the other unpleasant parts. Nothing lasts forever.

* * *

In August 2009, after the first batch of GEMFormulas' remedies and sprays were successfully made, I asked my step-son, Ryan, who was then a senior in college, to design the GEMFormulas' bottle labels and work on website graphics during his summer break. AriaRay helped me with our company logo.

I also started making videos about the products and distributing them on the internet to gain exposure and new customers. I began an email home study course. The first thirty-six lessons were written one at a time, every Saturday morning. I loved the regularity of this rhythm. For the most part, the information was dictated to me and then I edited it.

Editing raw transcripts has always been a critical and essential part of my process. Spoken language is far different than written language. Furthermore, to convey certain new information and bypass the limitations of my mind, my teachers would often give me the material circumspect. Only in the editing process did I gain enough knowledge to ask the right questions or pose the curiosities that would allow me to receive the details that would clarify a topic.

As I worked on creating the company and its educational materials during the day, at night I was learning how to maintain a dual consciousness. Inwardly I'd be bathing in the Light or having an inner experience with my gemstone teachers, and at the same time, I'd be outwardly transcribing the information I learned.

Sometimes the information would just pop into my awareness. Other times, I'd have conversations with Dr. Ay in his office, or listen in on planning meetings in the conference room with the Healing Council. I received insights about all aspects of my business. Every step of the way I was guided. Every GEMFormulas' product was preplanned and given to me. Trusting the steps the Healing Council gave me to take was easy because I had no prior experience of running a business. Following through, figuring out how to manifest the steps given, and managing the details was up to me and, eventually, also my staff.

In hindsight, I can see the wisdom of their plan: to set the foundation with the aura sprays, the gemstone necklaces, and the Gemstone Therapy Institute. Then the protocols I once glimpsed back in December, 2008, would be defined and outlined. Apparently, the Council wanted certified Gemstone Therapy practitioners in place before we began telling our story, which you're reading now.

The Council wanted to build a structure so that people who were interested in Gemstone Therapy had a variety of gemstone necklaces to choose from, practitioners they could visit for firsthand experience, e-Learning they could get started with right away, and curricula established for practitioner training. It was a miracle that the company survived long enough to manifest this vision in the preferred order.

I sometimes wonder if the Healing Council members inspired others to help us, too, because at every turn just the right people appeared. Experts in marketing, editing, and sales approached me offering their services—just as we needed them.

I also have to acknowledge my original customers. Many of them kept asking me if, in addition to the aura sprays, I would offer gemstone necklaces. I wrestled with the idea for months, for a lot of reasons. Among them, I didn't want my ex-husband to feel I was competing with him and I didn't want Bob to feel uncomfortable.

One evening after dinner, Bob and I were cleaning up the kitchen together, as usual. As I was drying the dishes, I was rattling off my list of pros and cons about offering my customers gemstone necklaces.

Bob was at the sink elbow-deep in soapy water. He handed me a plate and said, "Isa, if your customers want gemstones, why not give them gemstones?"

"You're okay with that?" I was busy drying as fast as he was washing.

"The gemstones were never the issue."

Bob's statement opened a door. I imagined talking to Dr. Ay about the idea, and lost in my daydream, a pile of wet dishes began to collect.

That night, I met Dr. Ay in his office. He was leaning out the window placing birdseed along the outside sill.

"I hear you are ready to offer gemstone necklaces," he said. Of course, he had heard my thoughts.

"It feels right."

"Then it's time we talked about symbiotic gemstones."

"Symbiotic gems?"

"Stones that catalyze, support, or strengthen the work of another gemstone," he said. He stepped gracefully toward his bench and sat down. I took my seat across from him as usual.

"A healing necklace must consist of one primary gemstone— to give the purpose of the necklace a focus. It must also contain its symbiotic partner in a much smaller amount."

"How come we never knew about this before?"

"I can give you an answer that may satisfy most who ask this same question, however, you should know a deeper truth."

I shifted my position on the bench. "Let's start with the easy answer."

"People's energetic needs have evolved since you first introduced Gemstone Therapy to the world in the 1980s. People are ready for a more sophisticated—and effective—way to experience gemstone necklaces."

"And the deeper reason?"

He turned to the window and looked at the pair of birds that had landed on the sill. "Where do you think knowledge of symbiotic gemstones came from?"

I shrugged. I didn't know.

"Yes. You know."

"Where did you learn about them?"

"Remember the Great Library?"

It seemed like a long time ago when I was there. I drifted back in my memory and recalled traveling into realms of even purer Light and then transcribing the information I had learned.

Suddenly it dawned on me.

I gripped the edge of the bench.

I had already learned the information! My heart failure had given me the opportunity to fulfill a karmic contract to collect knowledge of Gemstone Therapy. Had I not been revived, and allowed to bring out this information in this lifetime, I would have done so in the next.

The world needed it now.

Now when I meet the gemstone guardians inwardly, their presence helps me tune into those memories and that information. Often they embellish it and give it context. Always they teach me something new. I am always learning.

"Tell me, what did you learn about symbiotic relationships?" Dr. Ay asked.

"All good relationships are symbiotic," I said. "We serve each other. Even you and I have a symbiotic relationship. You and all the gemstone guardians support and catalyze my work with the gemstones and give me the strength and inspiration to continue. By sharing this information with others, I help you, too."

"And about symbiotic gemstones?"

"Usually only one or two types of gems provide symbiotic support."

I felt amazed. All I had to do was look within myself, access my memory banks, and there was the information I had learned during my near-death experience.

"Gemstone Therapy is all about healthy relationship," I said. "When necklaces that contain symbiotic gemstones are worn, they teach the body about good relationship. The body's intelligence centers see the perfect relationship between the gemstones and their symbiotes. They use this as a model for improving relationships among cells and organs inside the body, between the wearer and other people, and between the wearer and her Self."

I asked the library box for a tray of Agate spheres, strung temporarily into short strands. They appeared, and I arranged them into parallel lines.

"Notice your relationship with the Agate," I said to Dr. Ay.

I asked the library box for a strand of Citrine and placed it alongside the Agate.

I moved the Citrine closer to the Agate. The gems seemed attracted to each other, as though they were aware of each other's presence. I touched the gems together. "What do you notice now?"

"As soon as the symbiotic gemstones touch, the body recognizes them," Dr. Ay confirmed.

That's what I was feeling, too.

I moved the Agate and Cirine apart and then together a few times so that we could see for sure what was happening.

Dr. Ay nodded.

I set the Citrine atop the Agate, and the library box dissolved the hologram.

"Symbiotic gems also promote the balance of yin and yang in the body," Dr. Ay said. "Yin and yang represent the opposites in nature—and within ourselves as well. Opposites are balanced in a healthy person."

I realized the addition of symbiotic gems would also solve one of my own objections to sharing the gemstones. "Providing necklaces with symbiotic gems gives me something unique to offer," I said. I would not be competing with anyone.

"Your necklaces will also have clasps."

"All of them?"

"Go get that Leopardskin Jasper you haven't worn in years."

I hesitated. Did he actually want me to leave his office, return to my body, get out of bed, go downstairs and find the necklace? What if my connection to the inner worlds was lost?

"Sooner or later, you'll have to learn how to maintain your inner connection no matter what."

So I got up and retrieved the necklace. It was a continuous circle of gems, without a clasp.

I got back into bed.

"Now get some scissors."

I laughed as I got out of bed once again and went downstairs to the kitchen to get the scissors. Amazingly, I still felt Dr. Ay's presence. It felt as though he was standing next to me. I sat down at the kitchen table.

"What do you notice about the necklace?"

I tuned into its energies. "It feels as though it can't breathe."

"Cut it open."

I held the scissors between two beads, squeezed my eyes shut, and cut.

Whoosh! Instantly I felt a release of energy. I hadn't worn the necklace since the early 1990s. The gems had been holding this old energy for a long time. Now they were free.

"When a necklace's clasp is opened, it releases information and much of the unwanted energies the gemstones collect during use," Dr. Ay said. "Therapeutic-quality gemstone necklaces attract and sometimes absorb the unwanted and no-longer-needed energies of their wearers. As the gemstones uplift a person, a certain amount of dross is released. The wearer becomes free of it, but the gems pick it up. Opening the clasp releases some of it. Of course, the unwanted energies the gems collect still need to be cleared. If they aren't, they collect and the necklace becomes less and less effective. Once a necklace is cleared, its effectiveness is restored."

"I'm sure that's why single-gem necklaces without clasps tend to break so easily," I said. "Because they collect so much unwanted energies, they can't hold them anymore."

"Yes. That's exactly why that occurs. Originally you were told to use silk thread for this type of necklace to allow that to happen. It's a type of failsafe. Because your necklaces will have clasps, and be able to open, they can be strung with nylon. Nylon is stronger and more importantly, it is comprised of simple molecules that are practically inert energetically. Silk consists of complex protein molecules that some sensitive people will be unable to tolerate.

"Furthermore, you now have a way to completely clear the necklaces of any unwanted energies collected during use." Dr. Ay

241

showed me how to use the Energy Clearing spray on the Leopardskin Jasper. It looked more vital and alive than I'd ever seen it before. We then used the Electromagnetic Radiation Clearing Spray, because gemstones can pick up EMR. We finished the clearing by using the Seven-color Ray Diamond Spray, because gemstones have blueprints they can access too.

At a later meeting, Dr. Ay suggested that GEMFormulas' first necklace be Onyx with a single Ruby.

I had the combination strung. To my great joy, I found I could wear the necklace all day long—without it feeling heavy and uncomfortable. The symbiotic gem made the difference. While Onyx settles the energies within me that need settling, the Ruby lifts those that needed lifting. The body needs a flow in both directions to feel safe, grounded, and at home with itself.

The energies of the Ruby/Onyx necklace vitalize the first, or root, chakra. The red color ray, carried by Ruby, also nourishes this chakra. When this chakra is healthy, it helps propel a person forward on her life's path. How perfect—that's exactly what I needed.

* * *

By early 2010, the GEMFormulas business was moving forward with gusto. I was handling everything myself. What I needed next was some help. Could I afford it?

When Ryan graduated from college the summer of 2010, I asked him to work for GEMFormulas part-time. He and I managed every detail from gathering the gemstones and making the formulas, to filling orders and shipping them. By September of that year, he started working full-time. When we needed an extra hand, we hired Ryan's college roommate, Bill. Bill had a degree in communications and experience with customer service.

A humorous anecdote Ryan and I like to share that illustrates the company's growth involves a phone call I made to Ryan that autumn.

"We sold a necklace," I said to Ryan, "Tell Bill he can come to work tomorrow." Having made the sale, we could afford to pay him.

In early 2011, we asked Bill to work full time, and he soon became an integral part of our company. With Bill's help, Ryan could give more attention to the website, graphics, and video production.

Later that year, we needed another full-time helper. Because the company was still located in my home, we wanted to find someone whom we could trust and who would be compatible working with us in tight quarters. The story of how we hired Karie-anne illustrates how other decisions in our company are often made.

Since we couldn't think of anyone we knew who could help, I had to be patient and allow the spectrum of our need to magnetize its fulfillment. I also kept my eyes and ears open. One day, AriaRay mentioned that a girlfriend's father had lost his job. They were a family of four children. The thought occurred to me that his wife might be looking for work. When Karie-anne came to pick up her daughter at our house, she said something that made me think she might be open-minded enough to fit at GEMFormulas.

Later that day, I thought I'd call her and invite her to come for an interview.

"No," an inner nudge insisted. So I didn't. For the next few days, I kept checking for the rightness to call.

"No." "No." And "no," were my answers each time.

"But it feels right," I said.

"No."

Then one morning the inner voice came very clearly. "Call her now."

So I did.

Not only did Karie-anne have the experience we needed, she was intuitive, had a background in gemology, and loved crystals. After we hired her, she shared her side of the story. Had I called her any earlier than I did, she would have said "no." She needed the time to realize that she did in fact need to find work and to make peace with the idea of leaving her school-age kids at home during the day. Once she did this and had written her résumé, the universe answered her call and I was on the line.

In growing the company, I learned that taking steps forward went hand in hand with being patient and courageous. Needs and their fulfillments are two halves of a spectrum. One will draw the other in time, but you have to go beyond your comfort zone to identify the spectrum of need. Complacency and blind faith, although comfortable, don't manifest anything. I had to balance stepping forward with open-eyed trust and conviction.

Bob suggested I speak with one of our friends about the business. It was growing, and without having a business background, I wanted to make sure I was doing everything right. So one night we invited Chris and Debbie for dinner with the intention that Chris might share some insights afterward. He listened carefully. From the conversation that ensued, two pieces of advice stood out: To avoid costly overhead, keep the business at home until you can't stand it, and then keep it there longer. Second, to contact a mutual friend of ours, Joe, who was a retired small-business consultant.

For several months, Joe mentored me every Friday for an hour or so by phone, for free. Joe taught me about balance sheets, profit and loss statements, cash flow, the difference between employees and contract labor, and a long list of other basic business concepts. In time, we hired him and he came to our office regularly.

Kellan, who was then twelve, asked me how Joe was helping us.

I tried to explain.

She cut me off. "He's your ninja," she said.

"My what?"

She repeated. "He's your business ninja."

That's how Joe became our ninja. He has helped us through all types of situations, offering his extensive business experience and expertise. Best of all, he, as well as all the GEMFormulas' employees, have freed my time so that I can put it toward creatively moving the company forward with new information about the gemstones and Gemstone Therapy.

26

HOW THE NECKLACES HELPED ME

*P*ost-transplant, my health continuously provided opportunities to work with the gemstones and learn about what
they could do. Quite literally, I needed them as I was unable
to try other natural methods. My body was too sensitive to use
them. Any internal sensation, anything that "felt funny," could
make me feel panicky. Homeopathic remedies, essential oils, even
herbs, spicy foods, strong odors, or loud abrupt noises could send
me over the edge. Wearing gemstones over time has made me
feel stronger, more grounded, and secure. They've lessened my
super-sensitivities.

In 2012, I began to suffer from abdominal pain. My gastroenterologist was curious about this and after a few tests, he
decided it was blocked ducts in my liver. There was nothing he
could do without an invasive procedure. I felt desperate for an
alternative. That night, while lying in bed I opened a conversation with the Spirit of my Liver.

"I can't breathe," she said.

"What's wrong?"

"I'm suffocating."

"How can I help you?"

"Go ask Dr. Ay."

So I asked permission to visit, and the next thing I knew, I was standing next to him. He was replenishing the birdseed outside his window. This time, dozens of birds were flying around waiting for the food.

"It's time you remember more about the color rays," he said.

I strained my neck to look up at him.

"I want to."

"Good. Let's find out what color ray your liver is lacking."

Dr. Ay sat down on his bench, and I took my place across from him.

He reached into his pocket and drew out a small circle of gemstones. It consisted of one each of the color-ray bearing gemstones: Ruby, Carnelian, Yellow Sapphire, Emerald, Blue Sapphire, Indigo, and Amethyst, interspersed with a few beads of White Beryl.

He held the circle in such a way that he could test my liver with one color-ray gem at a time.

"Your liver is deficient in yellow."

He took out a decanter—which looked very much like the ones Hahn once used—and sprayed it above my liver. I didn't remember Hahn having used sprays; perhaps the idea had been too foreign and my memory missed that detail.

A curious yellow light illuminated the particles of mist as they rained down in front of me.

"What's that?" I asked.

"A color-ray spray."

This was the first I'd heard of them. I felt as though I was glimpsing the future—and indeed I was. It would be another year before I was given the gemstone mandalas to make them. I recognized the process of manifestation. First, I'd learn about or experience something inwardly, and in time I'd find a way to bring it into the physical world.

Dr. Ay retested my liver. Now it wanted green ray spray, and he gave it some. He tested my liver again. Now it wanted blue. My liver got some blue-ray spray. With each test and color spray application, I felt an energetic shift. My liver either relaxed, or opened, or seemed to reposition itself ever so slightly.

Each time Dr. Ay tested the color rays he always started with red and always tested all seven colors.

"Why bother testing the other colors after you get an answer?"

"To find out if two colors are needed."

He continued to test and correct my liver's colors a few more times and continued to get different answers until it settled on green three consecutive times.

"If a target area wants the same color three times in a row, it means it's time to wear a gemstone bearer of that color. The spray form cannot give the area a strong enough dose."

He handed me a necklace with Emerald and White Quartz. I was familiar with combining the color-ray gems with White Beryl as the symbiotic, because White Beryl's white light dissolves blockages in color ray flows. I'd never seen the gems combined with White Quartz. This gem is an opaque white stone comprised of microcrystalline quartz. It is also known as Quartzite.

"White Quartz will find the color-hungry places deep inside your body and deliver the Emerald's green ray there. You may prefer it as a symbiote, instead of White Beryl for the color ray stones when a target area is inside the body and when you expect the deficient color might change soon."

When I awoke the next morning, the pain had considerably lessened. In a few weeks, it was completely gone.

The next round of abdominal pain was in my kidneys. They ached deeply, both sides equally. I asked my general practitioner about it at a routine visit. After ruling out a list of possibilities, she suggested an MRI. When my urinalysis and blood work showed up as normal, I decided not to bother. I realized the symptoms weren't physically diagnosable, so I turned again to Dr. Ay for help.

This time, he suggested I wear a necklace we called My Ally, which was made of the gem formula Tree Agate, Light Green Aventurine, and White Quartz. I should also wear Bloodstone with Red Coral.

"Why did you choose gemstones for me, rather than test my color rays?" I asked.

"I didn't make that choice," he said. "I always ask your body's intelligence what it wants. These are the necklaces it chose. This combination hints that an infection is brewing somewhere in your body."

"My physical tests were negative for infection."

"Infections can exist at other levels of manifestation besides that of the physical body. Often they show up in the emotional body or at the molecular level. Wearing Bloodstone with Red Coral helps to address imbalances anywhere in the body and specifically at the molecular level."

"Can we test the color rays, too?" I asked.

"We shall. In fact, doing so will verify our suspicion about the infection."

He tested all seven colors. Yellow and green tested positive.

"We were right," he said. "When two colors test positive at any given point on the body, it means there's a foreign spectrum involved. One color reveals the most deficient color in the tissues' spectrum. The other color reveals the most deficient color in the spectrum of the foreign agent."

"You mean an infection."

"Foreign agents commonly manifest as an overgrowth of bacteria, virus, parasites, and fungus—what you might call infections—but are not limited to these."

He applied both yellow-ray spray and green-ray spray to the area where my kidneys were located. Then he proceeded to tell me more about color ray procedures, which became part of the Color Ray Protocol taught to students of the Gemstone Therapy Institute.

Soon enough, the kidney pain went away. The "foreign agents" as Dr. Ay called them were gone—although Dr. Ay would probably say they were back in balance with the rest of my body. We knew this because the area finally drew in just one color.

A year post-transplant, I transferred my care to a cardiology group closer to home and found a new cardiologist. I visited him every three months. Once when I walked into his office, the first thing he said was, "I see you have a skin cancer on your forehead."

Cancer is the top cause of death among transplant recipients. His statement would have sent chills down my spine except that his tone of voice was matter-of-fact, which helped me take the news in stride.

"I thought it was a viral sore."

His expression looked doubtful. He made an appointment for me with a dermatologist.

One of the blessings of the lesion was that it prompted me to ask for a Gemstone Therapy session from one of the practitioners I had certified through the Gemstone Therapy Institute. During the session, when it was time to state my intention, the words that came from my innermost Self surprised me. Instead of working directly with the lesion, my intention was to affirm the belief that "I have the capacity to heal myself." I had no idea that I doubted this. Gary performed the Belief Renewal Protocol to help anchor the belief into my physical reality. I can say with confidence that I now have a deep knowing that I am able to self-heal and renew.

Meanwhile, to soothe and vitalize the energies of my skin, I began wearing a necklace of White Flash Moonstone and Emerald. Nightly, I would test the lesion for color and correct the one that was most deficient. By this time, we had made the color-ray sprays and a replica of the color ray circle that Dr. Ay had used. Within a few weeks, the lesion was formally diagnosed and removed via MOH's surgery, leaving a nice new scar to add to my collection.

A month later, another skin cancer was removed near my collarbone. Each time something major happened with my health, my cardiologist lowered my doses of immuno-suppressant meds. After each adjustment, I felt much better. I'd feel less sick, less tired, and had far more energy.

My stomach was next in line to help me let go of something I didn't need. Even though I used my gemstone and color ray tools, the stomach pain persisted over several months and got progressively worse. I asked my gastroenterologist if I should increase my doses of a drug I was taking that was meant to protect my stomach from all the other meds.

"Do you have heartburn?" he asked when I came in to see him.

"No."

"Then I suggest you wean yourself off the drug."

Yes!

I was grateful to go of any medicine that wasn't helping me.

It was clear that my body was not going to tolerate any meds that it didn't need. Transplant patients walk a thin line between having enough immune-suppression to keep their new organ safe and having enough immunity to ward off disease and infection. This particular drug had nothing to do with immune-suppression. Without it, I felt again an increase in my vitality and the stomach pain disappeared.

Meanwhile, I was exercising more often and wearing gem-stone necklaces every day. My favorite at the time was Green Nephrite Jade with Prehnite simply because my body had a strong attraction to it. When I wore this necklace, I could feel my connective tissues finding new tone and relationship. It was as though the gems' energies were rearranging my body to accommodate the new reality of health I was reaching for.

Working with gems is different from working with herbs or medicines. We don't associate each gemstone with a particular disease or set of symptoms. There is not a gemstone "cure" for diabetes, backache, sore throat, skin rash, mental fuzziness, emotional distress, or broken heart. The gems address the underlying energetic causes and disharmonies associated with physical, emotional, and mental conditions. They also raise your body's vibrations. Therefore any therapeutic gemstone necklace you are attracted to can be beneficial. You cannot make a wrong choice.

Every morning I look at my collection of necklaces and, using my thoughts, I ask which ones among them would like to work with me that day.

Yes, I do talk to the gemstones—inwardly—and I do get replies, although usually not in words. Rather, I get nudges and knowing. Sometimes a necklace will pop into my thoughts, as though knocking at the door of my mind.

Then I test to be sure my body really wants it.

To do this, I'll hold the necklace in front of my heart, a little closer than arm's length. Slowly, I'll move the gemstones closer to my heart. If I feel a magnetic-like attraction that pulls the stones toward me, it means I could benefit from them. If I feel a cushion of energy that prevents me from moving the necklace closer to myself, then I know that I do not need these gemstones at this time.

Based on which gemstones my body wants, I gain an insight into what is going on. If my body wants Lapis Lazuli with Pyrite,

I know I need to work on the relationship between my heart, mind, and body. If a Golden Beryl necklace comes up, it suggests it's time to focus on the karmic implications of whatever is happening in my life at the time. If Spessartite with Rose Quartz and Rhodolite comes to my attention (a design I call "Sunray"), it tells me my endocrine system needs energetic support.

Besides their ability to nourish, gemstone energies are exceptional tools for clearing away the superfluous, to reveal what really matters. The most common type of unnecessary accumulation is like "dust on the furniture." Our body, emotions, memory, and mind typically collect non-essential energies. It's the natural effect of living in the physical world. Dust collects.

Energetic dust can cause everything from a sense of mental cloudiness and poor memory, to frustration, irritability, and lethargy. As the gems raise our vibrations, much of this unnecessary accumulation gradually falls away. A White Beryl/Turquoise necklace is especially good at dispersing it.

When you want energetic support from gemstones, you choose one based on their benefits and also your attraction. Your inner Self guides the affinity. If you have several necklaces, you might be drawn to wear one on a certain day and another on the next. Or both at the same time. If you are looking to choose one to wear long-term, your attraction will accommodate that intention, too.

When I began addressing the stomach pain, I was drawn to the color ray necklaces. The color ray that kept testing as deficient in my stomach was yellow. I used yellow-ray spray and began wearing rondel-shaped Citrine with White Beryl. The Citrine energies began unwinding a deep core tension. They also helped me see beyond my limitations. When I tuned in to what the gems were doing, I felt as though I was standing on the edge of a cliff. The cliff symbolized the limits of my present awareness, and I was seeing beyond it.

254

For the first time, I could apprehend the landscape of greater health. Once I saw, sensed, and felt it, I knew things were going to change physically too. I hoped they would soon—because my frequent and uncontrollable panic attacks were severely limiting me.

Since the transplant, I had two periods in which I was unable to drive due to uncontrollable anxiety that sometimes led to panic. The first occurred in 2005 right after the transplant. At that time, Bob suggested I talk with a psychologist.

I balked. I felt anxiety was something I should be able to control—if only I could focus my mind better. It also implied my spiritual tools weren't serving me as I thought they should. How could a spiritually-minded person succumb to panic? Where was my trust in God? Where was my sense of centeredness and inner peace? Why wasn't singing HU working as I thought it should?

Plus, I doubted Kitty could help. I was pleasantly surprised.

Kitty's office is a small room, wall-papered and pleasantly decorated. It's a haven of comfort, largely because of the atmosphere of safeness she creates. I fell into her soft white couch and explained my situation.

She knew exactly what was going on, "You're feeling anxiety because a part of your brain is still sending chemicals into your system as though the trauma you had experienced is still going on."

"So the anxiety is biochemical?"

"Yes. Your brain hasn't yet healed or adjusted to your new healthy circumstances."

So it wasn't a lack of spirituality.

Kitty was the first one to link my anxiety about driving with the fact that my donor had died in an automobile accident. This insight alone changed everything. If my donor died in a car, of course I would have an aversion to driving.

Over the next few weeks, I gradually drove more and more, until eventually I was able to drive AriaRay and Kellan to Maine during the summer of 2006.

The second period of anxiety started in November 2010.

To grow the GEMFormulas' business, I worked twelve to fourteen hours a day and balanced this by giving myself enough sleep. I'd usually not wake up until about 10:00 a.m., and on some days I needed to sleep a full twelve hours.

One evening, I was exhausted from a full day of work and hadn't yet eaten dinner. I had no way to cancel a prearranged parent-teacher conference. So, to keep my agreement with the teacher, I went. My daughter received a glowing report, and I left in good spirits.

On my way home, as I pulled up to a stop light, I started feeling palpitations and had trouble breathing. A policeman was driving in front of me and turned in the direction I was going in.

If the patrol car was a sign, did it mean I was safe?

Or was I in danger?

Sometimes signs can be so annoying.

I followed the officer past the emergency medical center and considered going there.

No, I decided. I will make it home and rest.

The patrol car remained in front of me.

The symptoms got worse.

When I could barely drive, I honked my horn, and the officer pulled over. By the time he got to my car door, I was ready to pass out. My heart was racing, my chest was so tight I could hardly breathe, and I was sure my I.C.D. was going to fire at any moment. The officer called Bob and the paramedics.

In some twist of time, I truly believed that I still had the I.C.D. unit in my chest. Every cell in my body was bracing itself for another round of v-tach and the storm of electrical shocks that would follow.

It was a nightmare come alive.

The paramedics came just as Bob pulled up.

"You don't have an I.C.D.," Bob repeated as they loaded me into the ambulance. "Your new heart is a healthy heart. It doesn't know what arrhythmia is."

Finally, the reality of my present circumstances filtered forward. I had experienced a panic attack of epic proportions. The doctors at the emergency room told me my heart was fine. I went home exhausted and humiliated.

I thought I'd already conquered anxiety and panic. Apparently not. The lessons in store would also chip away at my ego. For nearly three years, I was unable to drive. This meant relying on others to take me places. It also severely limited the experiences I could have with my children.

In an effort to be helpful, my mother sent me a newspaper article on anxiety. It painted a picture of people who didn't realize that anxiety was nature's way of keeping you motivated. Obviously, the author had never experienced a panic attack. Anxiety and panic are two very different things.

I have experienced the spectrum of anxiety. At one end, there's the excitement that keeps you up at night because you're in super-high gear, outflowing with creativity. You feel eager to keep the flow going and to complete a project at all costs. I also know what it's like to be unable to sleep due to anxiety about cash flow or some other aspect of the business. Then there's the anxiety I feel before giving a presentation. These feelings are a picnic compared to panic.

Panic is equally uncontrollable but also irrational and illogical. It engulfs you in a reality that makes no sense and smothers you in a black blanket of darkness so thick that it convinces you it's real. You cannot talk yourself out of it, nor think, feel, or command yourself back into control. Not only does it consume your thoughts and emotions, it can also take over your heart rate, breathing, muscles, digestive system, perspiration, bladder, and intestinal continence.

Almost as bad as a panic attack is the anxiety that comes when you're afraid that you're going to have a panic attack. This is what made driving impossible for me. Every time I got in the car to drive, I would experience some degree of panic or fear of panic.

Early on, I thought that overcoming the panic of driving was as simple as giving myself more driving practice. I'd go around the block and come right home. After a few times doing this successfully, I tried broadening my range. Bad idea. About two miles from my house, the panic struck. All I knew was that I needed to get home immediately and drove well over the speed limit to get there—in the rain. It wasn't safe. I needed far more than driving practice.

"The panic—it's all in your head." I could almost hear the admonishment.

But so is pain.

Neither is consciously controllable.

The patterns that prompted the panic were locked in my nervous system and somehow mysteriously tied with my new heart.

I began by asking my body which color ray gemstone would best support the healing of the anxiety. I learned it was the purple ray. In other words, purple was the most deficient color in the spectrum associated with the panic attacks. Therefore, if I wore a source of pure purple ray—Amethyst—my body would be flooded with that color. Purple would no longer be the most deficient color in the spectrum, and the experience of panic would therefore have to shift into something else.

Coincidentally, Amethyst is also the vitalizing gemstone for the nervous system. So I routinely wore Amethyst with its symbiotic White Beryl. White Beryl enhances all the color-ray-bearing gemstones because it clears blockages in the flows of color as they move both toward and away from the body.

Another necklace that was especially helpful for me is a design called Mountain Pose, which is made of therapeutic-quality Black Rhodonite and Onyx. It helped ground my emotions and gave me a sense of security, courage, and emotional foundation. I wore Mountain Pose with Amethyst/White Beryl whenever I practiced driving.

I also experimented by wearing a variety of other gemstone necklaces. Each one allowed me to approach my situation and learn about it from a different angle. One choice was Rose Quartz/Red Spinel. Rose Quartz helped me let go of some of the emotional energies stuck in my tissues, while its symbiotic, Red Spinel, allowed me to handle the release more gracefully because it would occur rhythmically.

I tried other methods too. My naturopath gave me a metabolic screening test and based on the results suggested I try a few supplements. By this time, I felt more comfortable trying new things. I wasn't as sensitive as before. The supplements helped a great deal to make my body feel more balanced and capable of handling unruly emotions. However, they didn't touch the panic.

I also received an interesting and very helpful treatment from an energy worker, who would remotely clear my aura while I was driving. I had the energy worker on speaker phone while I took the car down the road. When the panic started to surface, so too would anomalies in my energy field, which she then helped to correct. Meanwhile, I'd press the gemstone necklaces I was wearing against my chest to direct their energies into my body, where

I needed them most. Whenever I drove, I wore: Mountain Pose to keep my emotions settled and give me courage, Amethyst with White Beryl because purple was the color ray associated with the panicky feelings, and the Green Jade with Prehnite because it helped me keep my energies collected and under control.

Bob felt that my aversion to driving was Spirit's way of protecting me. Not from an accident but for self-preservation. I was giving all the energy I had to the business, and I had nothing left. If I started driving, I'd be tempted to go out more and this might mean drawing upon my energy reserves, which would compromise my health. Or I would have less time for the work, which at this point needed my full attention.

Up until 2013, my body had just enough energy to sit at a computer. I could not do much else. So I wrote articles, web-pages, video scripts, home study lessons, and the content of the foundation- and practitioner-level trainings. If I needed to lie down, I'd write in bed. It is possible that my inability to drive stemmed from physical exhaustion.

"You just want Bob to take care of you," one relative accused. "You're trying to control him."

"Is this true?" I asked Bob one night after dinner.

"I don't mind helping you," he said as he washed the dishes.

I wiped up the countertops. "I don't mean to control you."

"When God wants you to drive again, you will," he assured me. Then he took the sponge I was using, rinsed it out and invited me to go watch a movie with him in his man-cave.

I appreciated his confidence. Nonetheless, I ran myself over the coals trying to unearth reasons for the fear to help me understand myself and become a better person. Not being able to drive taught me to be humble, resourceful, grateful, and economical. If nothing else, it kept me at my computer, outpouring information on Gemstone Therapy.

Of all the things I uncovered in my psychological explorations about driving, foremost was the topic of trust. If I could trust God in every other department of my life, I could trust God in this one too. When it was time for me to drive again—when I was ready or when God was ready—I would.

One more treatment I tried is Phoenix Rising Yoga. A yoga therapist came by once a month to help me release the trauma from my tissues. We also did what I called Car Yoga, at my request. Beth, the therapist, would accompany me on car rides, and I'd drive until the panic started to rise. Then we would stop, and she would help me process the feelings and sensations.

This was when images of my donor's car accident began to come forward in full color.

We were driving on a lonely road in a forested area of my neighborhood. It was late morning, and the sun was streaming through the leaves. The beauty escaped me, however, as my attention was focused laser-like on keeping the panic at bay.

Suddenly, my self-control faltered.

Beth put her hand behind my heart and guided my breathing.

I pulled over to the side of the road, closed my eyes, and gave my full attention to the warmth of her hand on my back. She guided me to the edge of the experience, to the place where I had some control. I tried to calm down and find that place.

Suddenly, my inner vision filled with the image of an oncoming vehicle headed for my windshield. My body jumped. I heard the sound of metal crunching and glass shattering.

I realized that I had just witnessed, first-hand, my donor's fatal automobile accident.

27

CELLULAR MEMORIES

"Why do you do show me these things?" I asked my heart. I was by myself, sitting in the car, parked in my driveway. I spent time doing this almost every day, trying to feel more comfortable behind the wheel.

"Look what I experienced," she said.

"Yes, you've been showing it to me over and over again." The visions had been coming in ever greater detail.

"I want you to see."

"I see it," I replied. "It was horrific, but a miracle because you lived through it. You lived to tell about it, to remember it. To keep the experience alive." I tried to help my heart reframe the tragedy into an experience of success and survival.

In doing so, I realized that my heart was being badgered by cellular memories. These are the memories of events and histories that the cells store independently of the brain. If someone else's organ is now inside your body, its cellular memories will be there too.

Anyone who has endured significant trauma knows what cellular memories are. As much as you try to resolve and forget, your body won't let you. When faced with certain triggers, your body reacts and pours hormones into your bloodstream that stimulate fear, anxiety, or the visual replay of a haunting experience.

Cellular memories are like sentinels that never rest. When something happens that resembles the original trauma even remotely, cellular memories advance in full force, replaying the scenes that created them. Cellular memories can take total control, leaving the mind helpless and disconnected.

For me, cellular memories were the root of my post-traumatic stress, panic attacks, and the vivid memories of my donor's life-ending event. Not only did I have my heart's cellular memories of the car accident, I was also dealing with my body's cellular memories of the heart failure and the firing of my I.C.D.

Why won't the cells let go these memories? Because they consider a traumatic event too important to forget. The panic-stricken body believes that trauma equals important. If an event is traumatic, it must harbor a significant life lesson or information that must be retained for self-protection or self-preservation.

The body says, "I must remember this at all costs." And the cells fulfill that responsibility.

Cellular memories tormented me from November 2010 through the summer of 2013. Driving terrified me. Any resemblance of faintness, lightheadedness, quickened pulse, tightness of chest, palpitations, or hot flashes that I might experience in the car would cascade into panic. My skin would get prickly, my heart would race, my mind would shut off and rationality would evaporate. Images of a car accident would flash into my awareness, leaving me frozen in terror.

I remembered shattered glass piercing my face and body. The taste of blood. I sensed I had died instantly, except my heart was somehow protected, probably by the airbag?

As you may have noticed, I just told you about "my" car accident.

I began to remember and speak about my donor's experience in the first person. Sometimes I would talk about "our" accident and when "we" died in the crash. This felt natural. If anything, it signaled the transplant had worked. My heart had successfully blended with the rest of my body so well that she and I were one. So it was indeed quite true: we had these memories, and we needed to find peace with them.

One thing I had to work out was the question: what is the difference between my spiritual heart and my physical one? I've always looked to my heart for guidance and direction. With a new physical heart, is this guidance and direction my own? Is it meant for me or for my donor?

I learned that the physical heart is completely different than the spirit of the heart, which is the intelligence that gives you guidance and direction.

As I've said before, each organ has its own spirit, its own intelligence. The ancient Chinese had a special name for the heart spirit. They called it Shen. When my native heart was removed, its spirit left—but it did not have to. I know this because I had to consciously call back, or retrieve, my native Shen. This occurred early on in my healing process with the help of my craniosacral therapist. It was a significant turning point in helping me become more integrated and feeling more like "myself."

Does my donor's spirit live within me? No. I'm clear she passed into the heavenly worlds. I saw her go there. Yet, somehow I've inherited her Shen.

Both my native Shen and my new heart's Shen share space within me. They've learned to get along and support each other.

I am able to interact better with my Shen and my donor's Shen ever since they began to appear in animal form. My native Shen looks like a German Shepherd, who's faithful, devoted, and often on guard. The spirit of my new heart has manifested as a smaller dog. She's blonde, long-haired, and playful.

When I'm working at my computer, both dogs curl up and sleep peacefully. When I travel, the little one pokes her head out of my heart and rests her front paws on top of it—as though leaning out the window of a car. Her tail wags, her tongue laps, and her ears flap in the wind. She's as happy as can be. She's always excited about where we are going.

"To the swimming pool?" she asks. "Yes! We love to swim."

"To the office? Yes! We love to play with the gemstones."

"Home again? Yes! Let's go see Bob and do some writing."

On the highway in heavy traffic, she sometimes hides inside my heart, shaking and whimpering. The Shepherd barks. When I get anxious, I imagine petting my companions to reassure them that we'll be all right. They stop crying and barking and pant gently as we get through it together.

My relationship with these dogs is a close kinship. It's the friendship I share with my heart. We have traveled far together and are still learning so much. We are finding our strengths and overcoming our weaknesses. We are walking this healing journey and this gemstone journey together.

Clearly, it was not the Shen of my new heart that was initiating these flashbacks. They belonged to the cellular memories contained in the flesh of the new heart itself. In order to overcome the anxiety of driving, I had to fully accept these memories as my own and then work to reconcile them.

What happened to the memories of my native heart? They left when my native heart was removed. I don't remember having had certain negative emotions that people accuse me of once expressing. Jealousy? Rage? They're distant memories of feelings that others recount for me. Are they gone because the cells that housed them were removed with my native heart? Or were they purged during the emotional-body's heart transplant?

Obviously, the heart holds a great deal of memory.

It became apparent that the memories of our car accident were the reason I was unable to drive. I asked my heart spirits if they could become less reactive to the images. Would they please stop barking and running around in circles?

"Can we view the accident as though it happened to someone else, as though in a movie?" I asked.

"No, this isn't fiction. It really happened." Both my heart and my mind were adamant.

So much for that idea.

Another layer to resolve was revealed when I learned that my heart had not yet reset its clock to the present moment. It was still anticipating trauma associated with driving as though the accident was going to repeat itself every time I got behind the steering wheel.

To correct this, Dr. Ay showed me a Gemstone Therapy technique to evaluate whether areas of the body are present in the here and now—as they should be—or locked in the past or future. Then, how to perform the therapy to correct these temporal anomalies. So my experience taught me ways to help others, too. These techniques are now part of the Gemstone Therapy Institute advanced practitioner curricula.

Another tactic I tried was to fully accept the memories, rather than fighting them or trying to forget them. I sought them and consciously looked back in time to relive them, and to garner every detail I could. As a result, I came to terms with my donor's death and the horrific experience it must have been for the family. For a while, I grieved the loss. I now know absolutely that my donor is happy and free.

Due to a generous choice, a part of my donor lives within me. Life continued and either gave me, or unlocked within me, qualities I never before possessed or expressed. For one, I am now clearly a "type A" personality when before transplant, I was clearly "type B."

I like who I am and who we are. I like us together. I'm sure if I knew about my donor's personality, it would help me sort out what she gave me and what the experience itself unlocked. The transplant organization is very careful to keep details confidential. I may never know. Maybe it doesn't matter because what I've taken from this experience has made me a better person.

I do believe that heart recipients who experience new violent, destructive, or disturbing behaviors should be counseled about their donor's situation. I think this is essential to help a recipient sort out what is truly hers, what the transplant experience unlocked, and what cellular memories belong to the donor.

Transplant patients who suffer new and unhealthy behaviors should be treated by someone who can also comfortably converse with the spirit of the donated heart. I think this would help immensely.

Cellular memories? Yes, they are real. Do the cells in my hands remember holding the wheel of the car? No. Because they weren't there. Does my body remember some of the trauma my native heart felt? No, because that heart with all its memories is gone. My new heart held the memories of the accident and for a period of time insisted on projecting them like cinematic images into my mind's eye.

It took me a while to realize this next question. I asked my heart: "Why is it important to you to show me these memories?" The answer was a turning point.

"I don't want this to happen again."

My heart did not want to relieve the terror of being caught alone and alive in a body that was otherwise dead. My heart was trying to prevent me from driving because it wanted to avoid repeating that desperately cold and lonely experience.

268

To get some help, I made an appointment with a cognitive behavioral specialist. His wood paneled office was decorated with a single plant, his desk and chair, and the firm brown couch I sat upon. The spirit of his office was workmanlike—it was clear I'd be doing the work. I told him about my situation.

He suggested I reframe the accident. "Why not re-imagine it so that the accident did not occur?" he said. "That by some miracle the car swerved at just the right time to avoid impact?"

"I cannot do it," I said. "To re-imagine the accident not happening would mean that I am dead. Yet I am alive and I exist. It's an impossible conundrum. If I imagine my donor living through the accident, it means the heart inside my body is not there anymore."

My donor and I cannot both be alive together.

This is our fate. Yet in a very real way, we are always together: her heart is mine.

"What would happen if your heart let go of these memories?" the specialist suggested.

"You mean, if we forgot about the accident, what else would we inadvertently let go of?" This question led to another significant breakthrough: I realized my heart did not want to forget its native host. It remembered her by clinging to her death.

I asked the spirit of my heart if it could try recalling some of the good times they had. Letting go doesn't mean forgetting. It means shifting what you want to remember.

Was there something I too was not remembering? Was there something more I had not yet accepted? Another step on my gemstone journey that I had to take?

I would love to be able to pinpoint what finally erased my fear of driving. Instead, it was a gradual shift supported by many things including gemstones, exercise, fewer meds, a healing of my heart's cellular memories, and singing HU.

My cure also had something to do with frequent trips to New York City. For various reasons, including meetings with gemstone suppliers, attending concerts, taking campus tours, and visiting family, I found myself taking the train into the City every few months.

I fell in love with Manhattan and looked for excuses to go back. I can't tell you how much I enjoyed riding the subway around town, sitting in Central Park, trying various restaurants, window shopping, and visiting museums. The diversity, culture, and opportunities there inspire me.

When I was in New York, the jitteriness inside me was met by the edginess all around. Like a homeopathic medicine, in which like cures like, the intensity of the city counteracted the intensity of the anxiety. Fortunately, the cancelling-out effect persisted long after I returned home. Equally healing was the kinesthetic feeling of the train rumbling over the tracks, which was something I couldn't experience in my inner-world train.

One evening, riding home from the City, I sat in the last car. In our neighborhood, trains don't turn around, instead they go forward going one way and then backward going the other, or vice versa. On this next train's journey, the car I was sitting in would lead. This had been my goal all along—to move from the caboose to the engine.

While I'd been told my destiny was to move from the back to the front of the train, I never had the experience of walking through the train from one car to the next. No wonder, it wasn't about that. It was about taking a one-hundred-eighty degree turn.

This was a metaphor of my gemstone journey too. No longer was I going to trail behind or follow. I was going to lead.

28

TIME AGAIN FOR DIAMOND

O n May 22, 2015, I awoke with the terrible conviction that my life was about to change. With a profound sense of déjà vu, once again I scrambled to write down the dream. The words tumbled onto the page of my journal.

"It's time to start thinking about changing your…"

This time the five-letter word was unmistakable.

H O N O R.

I lay back down in bed, looked up at the ceiling, and listened to the sound of the ocean waves. We had rented a house on the ocean in Port Clyde, Maine, for a week-long company retreat. I was there to write and to do some high-altitude planning with my co-workers.

The dream was haunting, and my mind wrestled with it. It was time to start thinking about changing my honor? What the heck did that mean?

I got dressed and went outside to sit on the porch that overlooked the sea. Karie-anne and our newest employee, Melynda, were already enjoying the warm sunshine.

Seven months earlier, at our annual Gemstone Therapy retreat in October 2014, following a group discussion on Therapy Diamonds, Melynda and I had locked our eyes as a realization hit us at the same time.

"You're going to help me bring out the Diamond Program," I said.

"Yes, I am."

The truth held us in an extended moment of rapture.

Melynda had already put it out into the universe that she wanted to leave her job as a law professor in order to work with Gemstone Therapy. She'd had this realization when she attended a workshop of mine earlier that year. She felt she had found her destiny. How quickly the universe had responded.

It felt right to invite Melynda to our company. My inner pragmatist was silenced by inner knowingness. On the other hand, it felt as though everything was happening too fast. Was I ready to bring out the Diamond work once again? Could the company support another employee?

Over a year before, in January 2014, I was lying in bed, exhausted after a long day and ready to sleep when a beautiful voice asked me a question. It was a woman's voice. One that was familiar and comforting.

"Are you ready to share the Diamonds?"

"No."

I turned over onto my other side and away from the voice. I even covered my head with a pillow. How silly. This only meant it was easier to see through the darkness into the inner worlds.

My vision opened, and I saw the woman who had spoken. She was standing before me, petite, slender, and glowing.

Suddenly I remembered who she was, and I felt flushed. I thought about all the times when I was in the hospital living and reliving inner-world experiences. The angel in the Great Library and in the greenhouse with the butterflies, the one with the sparkles in her hair—of course. She was the Guardian of Diamond!

I felt a wave of unconditional love. The guardian was beaming. "Soon," she said.

"But not now."

I was certain I wasn't ready—and might never be. The razor's edge was too sharp; the risks too great. What if I couldn't maintain my balance and succumbed to the negative energies of a non-therapeutic diamond? What if others began applying non-therapeutic diamonds to themselves—or worse to others—and created magnificent anomalies in their auras?

"It will be different this time."

"How?"

"You are older, wiser, more yourself."

I liked to think so. I moved my head out from underneath my pillow. It was easier to breathe.

"Soon you will realize that you are not responsible if other people mistreat diamonds. You are only responsible for giving people the opportunity to use them wisely."

This would take some time to accept.

"How about at the upcoming Gemstone Therapy retreat?" she said.

"How about what?"

"You could give a short lecture about what Therapy Diamonds are and then let people experience what they feel like."

"I could do that." It was an easy step. We always like to give those who attended our retreats something special. This would be a unique opportunity for them.

As it turned out, everyone at the retreat loved the Diamond work. They seemed electrified by the Diamond energy, and excited about the potential of finding a closer relationship with their blueprints.

I did not expect our retreat guests to be so touched by Diamond or so moved. I didn't expect to be, either. That was when

Melynda and I connected and realized a potential future together at GEMFormulas.

A few weeks after the retreat, in November 2014, the Guardian of Diamond visited again before I fell asleep for the night.

"Maybe you should invite Melynda over to talk about her future role in your company."

It was a tactful suggestion. I still felt a great deal of personal resistance about sharing Therapy Diamonds again. A little chat and some future planning wouldn't hurt.

Melynda and I set a date.

A few nights later, the Diamond Guardian again visited me.

"If you're going to talk about diamonds, don't you think it would be nice to invite Linda?"

Linda had held the diamond torch after I left the work back in 1992. She taught a few Diamond Therapy workshops and continued to support those who had bought Therapy Diamonds the first time I'd brought them out. In 2009, she had been a close supporter when I re-introduced Gemstone Therapy and has continued to share the work both as a practitioner and teacher.

Linda's schedule was surprisingly clear on the days we had in mind.

"Yes, I can be there," she said.

January 2015 arrived. Linda, Melynda, and I sat around my old kitchen table. We had covered it with a tablecloth that matched our cherry-wood cabinets and the brickwork that framed them. The table was adjacent to our large kitchen window that overlooked the snow-covered lawn and the bird feeders that Bob religiously kept filled. It was the table where each of the GEMFormulas staff had once sat when the company was in our home. At the beginning, Ryan sat there. Then he shared it with Bill. When Bill moved his office into our living room, it was Karie-anne's, and also Lauren's desk space and then Sara's. Now it was ours.

We formally invited the presence of the Diamond Guardian to our meeting—although she was already there. In fact, it was she who was inviting us to move more deeply into the fountain of Diamond energy.

It felt so comfortable, and so right, that I dove in.

I felt the guardian's presence strongly, and she gave me a piece of diamond knowledge to share. As soon as our little group had completed our opening salutation, the words poured forth as though I'd known them all along.

"Seven-color-ray Diamonds have three attributes: fire, brilliance, and scintillation," I said. "The diamond industry acknowledges these physical characteristics. However, these terms also describe energetic benefits of diamonds."

Melynda began typing notes.

"Fire refers to the flashes of color that you see when you hold a diamond under certain lighting conditions."

I showed them my one-carat Therapy Diamond, and they looked for the flashes of fire. They were easy to see in my kitchen's natural lighting.

"These flashes of color are a physical attribute of diamond and not the seven healing rays that Therapy Diamonds carry. When applied a certain way, Therapy Diamonds remind the body of its color ray spectrums, then feed and correct the spectrums. Therapy Diamonds also have the unique ability to awaken our blueprint spectrums and then help them come forward into our lives to guide us."

The information was flowing, and I felt as though I couldn't speak it fast enough.

"A second attribute is brilliance. A diamond's brilliance is the effect of all its external and internal reflections of white light.

This physical characteristic of diamond relates to the energetic benefit called liquidity. When a Therapy Diamond is applied in a certain way, it spreads liquidity through the body. This increases communication, cooperation, and coherence among the liquidified areas."

I noticed Linda was taking notes, too.

"Let's open a shared Google document," I suggested, "so that we can each contribute to one set of notes."

When we were all on the same page, I continued. "The third attribute of diamond is scintillation. The jewelry industry defines this as the flashes of light and dark areas you see when the diamond, the light source, or the observer moves.

"Energetically, scintillation means something completely different. It is the natural fluctuation between matter and energy that atoms, and the tissues they comprise, should regularly experience. In a healthy body, scintillation occurs rhythmically. In areas that suffer with poor health, this fluctuation is often frozen. When a Therapy Diamond is applied in a certain way, it promotes scintillation in the body or in whatever area you want to target."

Linda and Melynda were fascinated by the concept of scintillation. It was based on a scientific observation that light can be observed as either a particle or a wave. In healthy tissue that same fluctuation should occur; it should rhythmically alternate between a state of matter and energy. Therapy Diamonds support that fluctuation and clear the blockages and stagnancies that inhibit it.

I applied my diamond to Linda and Melynda in such a way that they could experience what fire, brightness, and scintillation felt like.

"Scintillation feels as though I can switch gears more easily—on all levels," Melynda reported. "As though I'm able to see both sides of the coin or focus on either side at will."

Working with Therapy Diamonds put us in an expanded state. It felt remarkably freeing and inspiring.

"We are the Diamond," Melynda said.

"Diamond shifts our consciousness so that we can be aware of our blueprint truth," Linda added.

"People will get it," Melynda said.

"They already have," I said. "In the past few months, I've heard from people who want to begin working with Diamond again. I told them I wasn't ready."

"That's why we're here. To carry the work into the world and anchor it. So we can develop it further," Melynda said.

Around noon, the three of us prepared salad and some cooked vegetables. We continued our meeting while munching on crackers and goat cheese.

Linda looked at me and asked, "What do you think holds you back from being ready to share the diamond work?"

"I'm concerned about all the baggage from the past," I said. "What if it corrupts what we try to bring out this time?"

"We both have baggage," she agreed. Both hers and mine originated in the distant past, and while the details were hazy, she clearly recalled the feeling of having seen the negative side of diamonds.

I had too.

To help us overcome this hurdle, the Diamond Guardian gave me an idea for a procedure we could try.

"I have an idea that might help us let go of that baggage," I said. I outlined the steps we would take, and invited my co-workers to imagine the steps as I described them.

We took turns supporting each other through this technique in full two-hour sessions, where we practiced the steps of the Diamond Therapy Session Protocol that we also received. That afternoon, we worked on Melynda. Linda had her session after dinner, and I got mine the next day.

This procedure proved to have a powerful effect. We felt so liberated from our past that we decided this would be a keystone experience in our Diamond Therapy introductory workshops.

"We should also have a longer workshop," I said. "It should be long enough that participants could be immersed in diamond energy. They would have time to truly appreciate and respect what Therapy Diamonds were, learn how to work with them safely, and apply them therapeutically."

We all agreed that training would be a prerequisite for owning a Therapy Diamond. After all, you wouldn't expect to purchase powerful machinery without extensive training. Why not also give proper training to those who wanted to work with the Therapy Diamonds?

"When do you think we'll be ready to hold the first workshop?" Melynda asked.

"Soon," I said.

"As soon as possible," Linda added.

We all got out our calendars. Our year was already filling up with obligations. Mystically, it felt as though our meeting was opening a diamond portal, and we needed to fill it at the soonest possible opportunity. If we waited too long, unwanted energies might fill the opening instead.

We landed on the first week in March 2015. That was only eight weeks away, but everyone's schedule was open during that time.

"The weather could make things really interesting," Linda said. She would know. She lived in the mountains outside Boulder, Colorado.

Meanwhile, Karie-anne found a location for the workshop in Norfolk, Connecticut. "It's available on the dates you want," she said. "You could book the entire inn."

Our plans were falling into place effortlessly. Within hours after we decided to host our first Diamond workshop, we had dates and a location. Linda made a list of people who might be interested in attending. For this first workshop, we wanted to invite those who had already been called by Diamond and had expressed interest in the work.

We got on the phone and started calling people. "Yes, I'll come," someone said. "I'm in," said another. "I'll be there," said someone else. Nearly everyone we asked accepted our invitation.

While taking Linda back to the airport she became teary-eyed. "It's happening, Isa. We're actually going to do this. Whatever contract we had agreed to in the past, we're finally going to fulfill."

Yes, we were.

I had no idea that by the end of our meeting we would manifest a workshop. All along I had wondered if Diamond Therapy was going to be brought out again. Would it ever manifest? At times it felt nebulous. There is always free will, always the ability to say no. I'd said "no" plenty of times. This time, my heart was saying "yes." Never before had my heart felt so alive—nor had I felt so driven with purpose—not even with the gemstones.

The deep connection with Diamond that we shared washed over the both of us. We acknowledged the inner help we were getting too. It has always astounded us how much inner help is available—whether it's from our spiritual masters, the gemstone guardians, or those selfless anonymous helpers who show up during Gemstone Therapy sessions. All we need to do is acknowledge their presence.

The atmosphere of our meeting had been one of joyous celebration.

While it was clear the timing was right, in the weeks to follow, I felt as though our plans were as fragile as flower petals in a hard rain. We needed to protect the portal until the workshop was over. I asked the workshop participants not to share information about the rebirth of the diamond work until after the workshop. In fact, we weren't going to tell anyone about it.

The Law of Silence can provide a strong cloak of protection. I've learned this the hard way. I once shared a writing project with so many people that its energy dissipated. After working on the project more than a year, it lost its momentum and died.

March 2015 arrived and everything was going smoothly. The resistance began the day our guests were flying to Connecticut. A foot of snow had fallen, and a storm was headed our way. Flights were canceled or delayed. For me, what should have been a one-hour drive to Norfolk took over two-and-a-half hours. The snow was falling so hard, making my visibility so limited, that I took a wrong turn and got lost in the lonely mountains of western Connecticut.

I was fully aware how dangerous my situation was. It was dark, snowing, and cold. Most of the time I had no bars on my cell phone. The narrow, hilly roads were unplowed and sparsely populated. If not for the thick forest on either side of me, I wouldn't even know where the road was located.

"Spirit of my Nervous System, this is not the time to panic," I said aloud.

She agreed.

I called upon my spiritual guide for help and invited Rebazar to sit next to me in the front seat. I turned on a tape recording of the HU being sung by thousands of people and sang along myself. I imagined petting the dogs who personify the Spirits of my New and Native Hearts. I worked with Diamond in the protective way that the Guardian of Diamond had taught us in our January meeting. She had also shared a way to call upon others who also worked with Diamond. We formed an inner community that each of us nourished with our love and attention—and when necessary, like a bank account—could draw upon when needed.

It was a blessing I didn't feel any anxiety. It was a miracle I arrived safely.

When I pulled up into the driveway of the inn, our first group of guests had just arrived. How delightful it was to see them, bundled up in parkas and scarves and joyful to be there— as was I.

This first Diamond workshop hosted twelve people, including Linda, Melynda, and me. Twelve is the number associated with diamond. It is the number of wholeness, completeness, and universality. We saw it as a good sign.

When the workshop was over, the diamond energy felt anchored. It was time to announce our Diamond Therapy program.

Three months later, in May 2015, Melynda and Karie-anne were sitting with me on the porch beside the Atlantic Ocean. We had enjoyed three days of planning the structure of the GEMFormulas company so that it could have a well-defined matrix to fill in the coming years. It had been a productive company retreat.

Later that afternoon, after my co-workers had left for home, I found Bob sitting on the rocks next to the ocean. I didn't feel like sharing my dream about changing my honor. We sat in silence, listening to the sound of the water and being fed by it.

Our relationship has grown to this comfortable place where we don't need to say anything when nothing needs to be said. The ease we enjoy in each other's presence has grown deeper over the years. While it may not be politically correct to admit this, at times I feel more complete in his presence. More accurately, his spectrum completes mine, and vice versa. On most days, our colors are more beautiful together.

Sitting next to him, with our color rays nourishing each other, in the silence occupied by the sound of waves crashing upon rock, it was easier to examine my dream.

At first, my thoughts chewed on the dream. How do you change your honor? I didn't think one's honor could change. Maybe I heard the word incorrectly. Maybe it was another word beginning with H. Obviously the dream was telling me a change of some sort was coming. A part of me didn't want to know what it was because changes can be challenging.

When I stopped wrestling with the dream, I relaxed.

The waves of the incoming tide seemed to reach out to me. Were they trying to say something?

"All things either are alive, once-alive, or will one day support a life form." I heard the words in my head. This is what the Diamond Guardian had told me once, too.

Was this communication really coming from the ocean?

I looked over at a pile of gemstone necklaces, resting safely on a granite boulder. I had brought them to the rocks to take photographs of them by the sea.

They too, in their own way, were looking out over the water. Their relationship with the ocean reminded me of what I witnessed in Dr. Ay's office when we moved the Citrine close to the Agate. Clearly the gemstones and the ocean had a symbiotic relationship.

The meaning of my dream emerged. It was time to honor the gemstones newly.

"You're alive," I said inwardly to the gemstones sitting beside me. "I mean, you really are alive."

The realization was followed by a tremendous wave of gratitude that hit me like an oncoming wave and washed over me as though

I was one of the rocks. Emotion welled up.

The gratitude I was sensing was not mine—it was coming from the gemstones—and it felt powerful.

They were thanking me.

A customer once recounted his first experience with a gemstone necklace. When someone handed it to him, he felt a wave of energy move up his arm, "My God, it's alive!" Chris had exclaimed.

I agreed with him when he told me the story; however, it wasn't until this moment that I realized how very much alive gemstones are.

Suddenly, the gemstones became more than tools. They became my co-workers. My partners in my life experience. When I wear them, we enter a symbiotic relationship. The more I honor them, the more I can hear them and allow them to help me. Thus they fulfill their mission too.

I tell people: "When you apply gemstones in the aura, the body's energy recognizes them and moves them so that the gems' energies can go wherever they are needed most." While I sensed an intelligence behind the gemstones, I preferred to attribute their movement to the body's intelligence.

Now I realized something more was going on. The gemstones recognize our energies—and how harmonious they are or are not—perhaps better than we do. Their consciousness works with ours in a symbiotic relationship that heals us and heals them, too.

This new understanding was a transplant of a different sort. My rigid, self-centered attitude about what constituted consciousness was being washed away by the pounding waves and replaced by something softer, more accepting, and a lot closer to the truth.

I remember back in grade school when we learned what constituted life. To be alive, a thing had to have all the attributes of a human being. How arrogant this definition was, I realized. After all, if my tropical fish had intelligence and could express love, why not also gemstones?

If I was going to bring out the Diamond Program and step up to a higher level of integrity, I had to change the way I honored them and all Earth's minerals. I felt that I already honored the life-giving energy within them. Now I was being asked to honor their intelligence and life—wait—it was more than that. I was being asked to honor life itself. In all its forms and manifestations.

Every life form may express its consciousness differently— no one way is higher or lower than another, better or worse. All life forms have unique lessons and experiences, and all stand equally before God.

I looked out at the horizon where sea met sky. I realized that honoring the gemstones' intelligence and their unique way of expressing life is a first step toward our own evolution as citizens of the universe. As we reach out into space, we may encounter new life forms that may be very different than our own—and far more intelligent. If we cannot recognize them, why would they pay us any attention?

The tide had risen to the point where the ocean spray now splashed my feet. I acknowledged the ocean's consciousness, too. I felt a growing kinship with it and the rocks I sat upon. I sensed the connection between myself, the gemstones, and the Atlantic and that this connection included all things into infinity.

"We are all connected," I said aloud.

"Pardon me?" Bob said. He thought I was talking to him.

"I was just talking to the ocean." I'm weird, remember?

"Okay." He loves me anyway.

I stood up to walk along the seaside, stepping from one

boulder to the next, toward the lighthouse where Bob had proposed marriage eight years earlier.

I heard a voice speaking to me telepathically. "Honor yourself. Honor the life around you. Life supports life."

"Who's there?" I asked inwardly.

This voice had no distinct owner. It was a different sort of voice. It came from no one direction, no source in particular. Instead, it came from everywhere, as though all the atoms in the air around me and the ocean before me were speaking to me in one voice. This was the voice of life itself.

It was time to honor myself, too.

For whatever reason, life had chosen me to continue to walk this Earth in this lifetime. For some reason, this Soul who I am has a contract to teach people about new healing modalities. In this lifetime, it's Diamond and Gemstone Therapy. It is what I'm meant to do.

The wind had picked up, and the waters now looked choppy. I made sure my feet were firmly planted on the boulders, and I faced the sea. The wind blew softly across my skin.

Then, I reexamined my core beliefs—which is something I like to do when I'm feeling too much change happening much too fast.

Regarding Gemstone Therapy: I believe it has an important role in alternative medicine. The energies that comprise our being require as much support, nourishment, and care as our body does. Working with stones makes this easy. Furthermore, I believe that Therapy Diamonds and gemstones will play a critical role in the survival of humanity into the next century. We need them.

Regarding my changing honor: I believe that honoring myself makes me a more humble human being, more in touch with myself and all life. To express that honor, I am destined to share the Diamond Program once again.

Regarding that program: I believe that I am finally ready.

Regarding my heart: I've become comfortable and secure in our relationship. Thanks to her and to my native heart, I know for sure that life continues on the other side. I've seen it. I've experienced it. I chose to come back to this lifetime and was granted my wish. I will be here for as long as I'm needed. Then I'll gladly go wherever life wants me to experience itself next.

Maybe at the conclusion of my existence here, when I'm on the other side for good, I'll have a chance to meet the Soul who gave me my heart and a second chance at life. I would enjoy that.

Upon my death, the spirits of my old and new heart, in puppy form, will spring out, free at last. The little one will run toward my donor—tail wagging, ears flapping—and leap into her arms, returning home at last. The German Shepherd will remain by my side.

My donor and I will recognize each other from afar.

We will walk toward each other. We will embrace. This time, she won't pass through me.

Holding hands, we will step back to look into each other's eyes and smile and laugh. We'll have a lot to share and plenty of time to do it. Then she and I will walk hand in hand, back into the Light, together.

And the spirits of our hearts will play and run along beside us.

* * *

Thank you for reading my story.

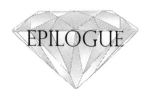

EPILOGUE

I enjoy watching movies.

I come home from work, have dinner (Bob usually prepares the meal for us), and then go to my desk to write. Frequently, Bob comes to visit a few hours later.

"Want to watch some baseball or a movie?"

"Sure!"

He helps me stay balanced.

My favorite part of watching movies (besides his company) is seeing the extras. The deleted scenes that didn't survive careful editing give me keen insight into what the director had in mind.

I, too, have a collection of outtakes and deleted scenes. They're a random assortment of anecdotes and experiences that didn't fit the structure of this book. May they serve to give you a better idea of what my journey of heart transplant was like. Visit *www.isabellemorton.com*, and click on *Accepting Destiny Outtakes and Deleted Scenes*. To access the file, which is reserved for readers of this book, use the password "MORE".

ACKNOWLEDGEMENTS

*O*ne of the benefits of writing a memoir is that it gives me the opportunity to publicly express the heartfelt gratitude I feel for the special people in my life who have loved me, supported me, and helped me grow.

Gratitude first to my mother and father, who love me no matter what: Virginia Bedesem and William Bedesem. Thank you also to my step-mom, Fenella Bedesem, and also my mother-in-law Mary Lou Widman. My brothers, Lt. Col. Paul Bedesem and his wife Kathy; and Lt. Col. Brian Bedesem and his wife Liz. Thank you for your love and support and for being there.

My children, you deserve deepest respect for all you experienced as a result of the choices I made as well as the ones I could not control. Emily, Eleena, Eranel, AriaRay, and Kellan, I love you more than you'll ever know. Thank you for loving me back.

Thank you Mary Carroll Moore for helping me make this book the best it could be. It wouldn't be what it is without you. Melynda Barnhart and Elke Rhomberg, thank you for reading early versions and sharing meaningful feedback. Mariana DiRaimo, thank you for your careful line editing. AriaRay Brown, thank you for the brainstorming session that resulted in the title of this book. Thank you Robin McBride for the beautiful typesetting and cover design. You made the book come alive! Thank you Gabrielle J. Selle, Esquire, my literary attorney, for your counsel. Thank you Susan Harrow for helping us plan our marketing and book publicity.

Thank you to the medical staff who assisted me on my journey; you are the best. I cannot name all the doctors, fellows, nurses, aides, and other staff because you were so many. I was able to develop a relationship with a few of my doctors and you deserve special thanks for being brilliant in your field as well as going beyond the call of duty for me on many occasions: Dr. Anthony Lasala MD, Dr. Jeffrey Kluger MD, Dr. Christopher Clyne MD, Dr. Anju Nohria MD, Dr. Gregory S. Couper MD, Dr. Karen Cadman MD, Dr. Laura Bony MD, and my current post-transplant cardiologist Dr. John Granquist MD.

Thank you Kim Meyer-Pelletier, my cranial-sacral therapist; Beth Wyatt, my Phoenix Rising yoga therapist; Kitty Ansaldi, APRN, psychiatric nurse practitioner; and Vicki Cashman, energy-worker extraordinaire.

Thank you to my neighbors Bonnie Brunell, and Jack and Lorraine Kreeger for being there and helping me when I needed you. Thank you Michael DiRaimo for the rides to rehab.

Thank you to the ambulance drivers who always got me there on time. Thank you to the hospital cleaning staff, who were always so cheerful and willing to share a smile.

While I was in the hospital awaiting my new heart, I received cards, flowers, books, poetry, goodies, and little gifts. A day didn't go by without there being something for me in the mail. My friends and family, I thought you would forget me, but you never did. I will never forget you either. I have kept all the cards you sent, wrapped in ribbon: Mom, Dad and Fenella, Paul, Brian; Mary Lou; Aunt Alma Hoder; Aunt Dolores Kelble and Uncle

Dick Kelble; Aunt Helen Walker and Uncle Lewis Walker; Aunt Vera Bean; Adriana Allen; Andy Kulick; Anne Barriere (thank you for the DVD you made of friends wishing me well!); Barbara Battey; Barbara Russo-Smith; Becca Anderson; Bert and Alita Blackburn; Brad and Diane Petersen (thank you for regularly sending me books to read. They were a welcome respite); Carol Serio; Carol Williams; Chris, Deb, Lauren, and Alex Chessari; Dan Schwartz, Deb Fuller (thank you for the comic strips!); Deonn Bunnell; Doreen and Sam Kasper; Dorothy Flagg; Emily Katz; Emma Laurence; Fred Lipsius; Gloria and Pete Brooks; Grace and Tom Bloomfield; Irene Salvatore; Ivan Anderson; Jack and Lorraine Kreeger; Jackie Flatow; Jamie and Lynne Fairley; Jan Hansen and Gary Goodell; Jean Giordano; Jill Morton; Jim Bennett; Joan Foberg; Joanne, Ron, Lauren, and Ronnie Missal; Joanne and Richard Wace; Joe and Nada Light (thank you also for the poetry); John and Ruth Cloonan; John Noonan; Kim Pelletier; Kim Briggs; Krystin Varela; Kurt Anderson; Lana Westgate; Linnie York and Craig Chessari; Lisa, Kevin, Leah, and Lauren Duran; Luanne and Bob Lawton (thank you for the socks and sweatshirt, I wore them every day); Marie and Glenn Andrew; MaryLou Widman; Matt and Connie Kresz; Michael Starkie and Christie Qu; Mike and MaeBeth DeLuca; Pat, Charley, and Melody Boyd; Patti and Steve Towhill; Peter Lucchese and Patti Lucchese; Richard Lawson; Rick Buell; Rick, Isabelle, Paul, and Amelia Duffy and Monique Regard; Ruth and Frank; Sebastian Correa; Sue and Bill Armstrong; Sue Crowley; Terri Cermola and Phil Hunter; Tony and Donna Lupinacci; Virginia from the nursing home; and Faye Ferris and everyone from my cardiac rehab class. If I have missed your name, please forgive me.

Randy Jacobs, Andy Kulick, and Fred Lipsius, thank you for visiting me often while I awaited my heart.

Thank you to my donor and donor family.

Thank you to the spirits of my organs, and especially the spirits of my hearts. Thank you to the spirit of the GEMFormulas company.

Thank you to the guardians of the gemstones for your willingness to share your knowledge and forgive my ignorance. Thank you to the inner-world Diamond and Gemstone Therapy teachers and assistants. It always amazes me how willing you are to help.

Thank you David for keeping the work alive all these years, and helping me get back on track. I have always admired your generosity. Thank you for raising our children. Thank you Stephen Brown for sharing my journey through the 1990s.

Thank you Ron Heacock for giving me a copy of *In My Soul I Am Free*. Thank you Bill and Kathy Hall for your friendship. Thank you Dr. Michael Crouch and Karen Kolczak for being good friends and supportive listeners while I manifested my dream. Thank you Dr. Elizabeth Hooker for watching my back.

Thank you to Linda Lile, our first Gemstone Therapy Institute instructor, for your tremendous patience, trust, and support. Special gratitude to the first ten active certified Gemstone Therapy practitioners: Herbert Wheeler, Robyn Arrington, Stephanie O'Dell, Marjorie Hill, Debra Kraft, Gary Wright, Debra Medley, Joan Lunney, Harriet Olmstead and Dr. Cari Nyland. (Listed in order of their certification.) Thank you for the respect you give the gemstones, and your unfailing understanding and support. I like to think we make a good team.

Thank you to all my GEMFormulas' customers and Gemstone Therapy Institute students. Without your interest in the work, my life would have no purpose. You have a special place in my heart.

Thank you to my staff at GEMFormulas for keeping the ship moving forward while I spend time writing and teaching: Ryan

Morton, Bill Young, Karie-anne Everlith, Joe Light, Sara DePietro, Renee Garceau, and Melynda Barnhart. Thank you Fadil Berisha for your photography.

Bob, you are my rock, husband, and friend. You understand me more than anyone. You have taught me what it means to give companionship, kindness, and service. I feel blessed to spend the rest of my life sharing my gratitude with you.

Gratitude beyond words to my spiritual master, Harold Klemp, and his co-workers, especially Rebazar Tarzs. You really are always with me.

EXPERIENCE AND LEARN

Looking back on my experiences, I feel blessed to have had them. What an extraordinary opportunity I've had to learn about the healing potential of gemstomes. Thanks to my staff, I am able to provide you with a variety of ways that you too can learn and experience Gemstone Therapy.

Gemstone necklaces, bracelets, and earrings

GEMFormulas' aura sprays

E-learning and home-study courses

Workshops on Gemstone Therapy and Diamond Therapy

Gemstone Therapy Practitioner certification

Diamond Therapy Practitioner certification

The opportunity to receive Gemstone Therapy remotely
or in person by certified Gemstone Therapy and
Diamond Therapy Practitioners and interns

Gemstone Therapy Retreats—where you enjoy daily
intensive Diamond and Gemstone Therapy in
a safe and supportive setting

Visit us at *www.GEMFormulas.com* for details
and to sign up for our newsletter.

Here is a poem composed for me while I was awaiting my new heart:

Whispering sounds of HU
Bathe her body like gentle water
Flowing over forest waterfalls.

Let Sound surround her,
Enter her spiritual space,
Background music for all life.

Friends hold her in their daily HU
Inspired by her courage and
Knowing all bodies are cubicles for
Spiritual Challenges.

—by Nada Light
December 20, 2004

Made in the USA
San Bernardino, CA
20 December 2019